Neuropsychology of Stuttering

Neuropsychology of Stuttering

Edited by Einer Boberg

The University of Alberta Press

First published by
The University of Alberta Press
141 Athabasca Hall
Edmonton, Alberta
Canada T6G 2E8

Copyright © The University of Alberta Press 1993

ISBN 0-88864-239-3

Canadian Cataloguing in Publication Data

Main entry under title:

Neuropsychology of stuttering

Papers presented at the 3rd Banff International
Conference on Stuttering, held 1989.
Includes bibliographical references
ISBN 0-88864-239-3

1. Stuttering—Congresses. 2. Neuropsychology—Congresses.
I. Boberg, Einer. II. Banff International Conference on Stuttering (3rd : 1989)
RC424.N47 1993   616.85′54   C93-091133-4

Printed on acid-free paper.

Printed and bound in Canada by
D.W. Friesens & Sons Ltd., Altona, Manitoba, Canada

This book is dedicated to my colleagues
in stuttering treatment and research for their inspiration
and encouragement throughout my career, especially

Richard Martin
William Perkins
Hugo Gregory

Contents

Oliver Bloodstein

Foreword

Many active researchers in stuttering see neuropsychology as the most likely area for obtaining new insights into the nature of this baffling disorder. After decades of unverified theories and equivocal research findings based on the premise that stuttering is wholly learned behavior, the premise has grown stale. Viewpoints with a physiological orientation have that invigorating aura of promise that new departures almost always bring with them.

This is by no means the first time that researchers have concerned themselves with the stutterer's physical constitution. From about 1925 to 1945 there was intensive investigation of the neuromuscular organization, cardiovascular functioning, biochemistry, and motor coordination of stutterers. Little came of this research. It was plagued by primitive instrumentation and questionable procedures. One by one, enthusiastic reports of significant findings were eventually found to be due to such errors as the failure to test subjects under basal conditions, the use of previously established norms in place of control groups, or statistical analyses in which N's were inflated by the use of numbers of measures rather than numbers of subjects. A half century has passed since this early effort petered out in confusion. We are now in possession of far better instrumentation, and the conduct of research in speech pathology has become a science in itself. There are grounds for belief that the neurophysiological findings being reported presently may prove to have a firm basis in fact.

The clinical implications of this new development are as yet difficult to foresee. But we should not lose sight of the fact that the research has already had one practical result of incalculable benefit. It is destined to liberate stutterers and their parents from the stigma which many of them felt when stuttering was confidently assumed to be due to a failed home environment or to be a wholly learned reaction that a person should be able to unlearn by practicing hard enough.

It is unfortunate that positive developments must often have unfavorable side effects. The possibility that stuttering may frequently have a subtle neurophysiological component lends itself all too easily to the assumption that it is an "organic" disorder. Already the news media, with their hunger for the simple and dramatic, are spreading the word that stuttering is a "medical" problem. The facts militate against such a gross oversimplification. For one thing, the evidence for the role of environment in stuttering cannot be denied. There is no other way to account for the cases of discordance for the disorder in identical twins. And as Kenneth Kidd has shown, in order to explain the observed familial distribution of stuttering cases, we must assume that environmental influences interact with genes to cause the problem. Another fact that we cannot ignore is that the neuropsychological peculiarities that have been reported to characterize stutterers as groups are not present in all individuals and are found in some nonstutterers. The peculiarities may not be involved in the etiology of stuttering in any simple, direct way. Finally, it is generally acknowledged that, whatever the cause of stuttering, the preponderance of its observable phenomena is the product of learning. It is unnecessary to review here the mass of relevant observations. One has only to remember that a stutterer blocking on one word may immediately articulate a substitute with ease; or that in repeated readings of a passage, a stutterer tends to have difficulty with the same words, and that these words differ markedly from subject to subject.

In short, stuttering is not apt to give up its secret to such conventional categories of scientific approach as are labeled "organic," "functional," "psychological," or "neurological." The perception has been growing for some time that we need new mental sets even more than new theories or laboratory devices. Major scientific discoveries are often made at the boundaries between old disciplines when researchers break down barriers to create new disciplines such as biochemistry or molecular biology. It seems altogether likely that when we find the explanations we are looking for, it will be in some such hybrid field. It is not beyond belief that we will find some of them in the neuropsychology of stuttering.

Preface

Those of us who work with and try to understand stuttering are experiencing déjà vu. About 60 years ago Orton and Travis sought to demonstrate that stuttering was related to abnormal brain function. The Third Banff Conference on the Neuropsychology of Stuttering in 1989 focused once again on stuttering and abnormal brain function.

After the provocative beginnings of brain function research pioneered by Orton and Travis most speech pathologists abandoned the search for causal factors within the person. Led by Wendell Johnson and his colleagues at the University of Iowa, researchers sought instead potent factors in the environment which could account for the onset of stuttering. Their research mirrored efforts in many other disciplines at mid-century to find environmental explanations for human conditions as disparate as autism, homosexuality and drug addictions.

By the end of the 1960s some researchers, not convinced by the environmental explanations, were determined to have another look inside the stutterer for neuropsychological and neurophysiological correlates of stuttering. With the advantages of new technology and the knowledge derived from developments in neuroscience, this new generation of researchers re-examined the earlier investigations and launched new studies in an effort to find the underlying basis for stuttering. By the late 1980s, since so many investigations had been completed and much data accumulated, it was logical for the Third

Banff International Conference on Stuttering to focus on neuropsychology and stuttering. Seven prominent scientists presented data,
interpretations and reactions to 90 keen participants from five coun-
tries. This book presents highlights of that conference.

Reports of experimental investigations by eminent clinical scientists are presented in the first four chapters of the book. Catherine
Mateer's paper provides a framework in which to interpret experimental data and consider their implications for stuttering. She
describes brain development and cerebral asymmetries, the neural
bases of language organization and the patterns that emerge in individuals who demonstrate atypical language lateralization. Dr.
Mateer also points out potential relationships between these phenomena and the dysfluency research.

Walter Moore traces the development of neuropsychological
research from the early work of Orton and Travis, through the
decline of interest at mid-century in favour of environmental explanations of stuttering and the resurgence of this research in the late
1960s. Dr. Moore describes the advantages and disadvantages of different electrophysiological procedures and then reports some of his
own investigations of hemispheric processing.

In the third chapter William Webster begins by stating the
assumptions that underlie his work: 1) there is a biological basis to
stuttering; 2) the biological basis is neurological; 3) we can learn
about brain mechanisms associated with speech motor control
through the study of the control of other motoric processes. Dr. Webster then describes his extensive research on hand movements in
people who stutter, what those hand movements reveal about the
mechanism of speech motor control in stutterers and some implications for the treatment of stuttering.

Lorne Yeudall and his research team submitted their chapter for
publication after the conference as he was unable to present it at the
conference. Dr. Yeudall describes an investigation of 17 stutterers
which examined variability in subjects pertaining to severity, results
from therapy and levels of involvement of different brain systems.
Theoretically, Yeudall and his colleagues view stuttering as a
dynamic interaction of brain systems, notably the cortical motor sys-

tems of the frontal lobes and associated subcortical structures, including the limbic system.

Richard Curlee and Roger Ingham present their critical views in separate chapters on the implications of current research for diagnosis and clinical management of stuttering. Their conclusions are provocative and led to lively and sometimes heated interchanges at the conference. This healthy debate, in the best of scientific traditions, should encourage clinical scientists to examine their own beliefs about the relationships of research data to what they believe about the nature of stuttering and what they do in their clinics.

In the final chapter, William Perkins, a senior scholar in the profession, presents a conceptual theory of the neural functions that underlie the cognitive, linguistic and behavioral characteristics of stuttering.

A special feature of the Conference was the opportunity for small group discussions following each presentation. Discussion leaders encouraged all group members to react critically to the papers presented and add comments based on their own experience and knowledge. Toward the end of this free-ranging, informal discussion each leader tried to crystallize the group 's comments into three or four carefully worded questions.

The questions presented by the discussion leaders, the speaker 's response to these and additional audience questions were recorded and have been transcribed from the audiotapes for inclusion in this book. Since there is often a substantial difference between a person 's use of language when participating in a free-wheeling, spontaneous discussion and the more formal written style, it was necessary to edit this material to communicate accurately the information contained in the exchanges while preserving the speaker 's unique style.

In the epilogue, three of the discussion leaders comment on the papers and discussions presented at the Conference.

New directions and developments in a clinical field such as stuttering are often greeted with a mixture of excitement and skepticism. Proponents believe that the methodology and information base of neuropsychology will expand the basis for understanding the nature of stuttering and will also lead to advances in assessment and treat-

ment. Critics warn of the dangers of premature inferences and speculation and see few if any implications for assessment and treatment
in the published research.

This book provides a unique opportunity for scientists, clinicians
and students to share the enthusiasm, excitement and conflict that
exist on this frontier of stuttering research. Readers are encouraged
to examine the methodology and results of these experimental investigations, consider the critiques and then determine for themselves
the potential contributions of neuropsychology to our continuing
quest to improve our understanding and treatment of stuttering.

Acknowledgements

Many people have contributed to the planning of the conference and the production of this book. My interest in the neuropsychology of stuttering was kindled by long discussions with three eminent clinical scientists: Walter Moore, William Webster and Lorne Yeudall. I appreciate the enormous importance of their work to those of us who are fascinated by stuttering.

The following agencies provided financial and other support which made the conference possible: The Alberta Heritage Foundation for Medical Research; the Institute for Stuttering Treatment and Research; and the Division of Continuing Medical Education at the University of Alberta. I thank them all for their help and am particularly grateful to Olga Nixon and her staff in the Division of Continuing Medical Education for handling the administrative details with such efficiency. The exceptional cooperation and support from the staff at the Banff Conference Centre were also much valued by the conference participants.

I thank the conference discussion leaders for creating an atmosphere in which ideas and information could be exchanged freely. They had the extraordinarily difficult task of guiding the frequently animated discussions and extracting pertinent questions from the barrage of comments. In addition I thank the conference assistants who chaired the sessions, directed the exercise breaks and audiotaped the question period with the speakers. Special thanks go to Vicki Ross, who transcribed the question period discussions from the audiotapes and typed large sections of the manuscript, and to Laura Manz and Julia Boberg who assisted in the final preparation of the manuscript. I also express my warm appreciation to the University of Alberta Press for undertaking to publish this book.

My deepest appreciation is extended to the authors for their generous contribution towards both the conference and this book. The publication of these papers and discussions will enable many readers to benefit from the authors' extensive research and clinical experience.

Finally, I want to thank Oliver Bloodstein, another senior scholar, for providing a broad perspective on recent developments in stuttering.

Contributors

Oliver Bloodstein is a professor emeritus at the Speech and Hearing Centre, Brooklyn College of CUNY, New York.

Einer Boberg is a professor in the Department of Speech Pathology and Audiology, University of Alberta in Edmonton and executive director of the Institute for Stuttering Treatment and Research.

Ken Burk is a professor in the Department of Communicative Disorders and Sciences at Wichita State University in Kansas.

Anthony Caruso is a professor in the Department of Speech Pathology and Audiology at Kent State University in Ohio.

Richard F. Curlee is a professor in the Department of Speech and Hearing Sciences, University of Arizona in Tucson.

Orestes Fedora is a psychologist at the Clinical Diagnostics and Research Centre, Alberta Hopsital Edmonton.

Robert Kroll is the director of the Speech Pathology Department at the Clarke Institute in Toronto, Ontario.

John C. Lind is a quantitative psychologist specializing in experimental design and statistics at Alberta Hospital Edmonton and adjunct professor at the University of Alberta.

Hugo Gregory is a professor emeritus in the Department of Communicative Disorders, Northwestern University in Evanston, Illinois.

Laura Manz was the clinical coordinator at the Institute for Stuttering Treatment and Research and is currently the Supervisor, Speech-Language-Hearing Program, Watoka Health Unit, Wetaskiwin, Alberta.

Catherine Mateer is a professor in the Department of Speech and Hearing Sciences and the Department of Neurological Sciences at the University of Washington in Seattle.

Walter H. Moore is a professor in the Department of Communicative Disorders at California State University in Long Beach.

Megan Neilson is a clinical investigator at the Clinical Research Unit for Anxiety Disorders at the University of New South Wales in Darlinghurst, Australia.

William H. Perkins is director of the Stuttering Center in Los Angeles and a professor emeritus at the University of Southern California.

Cathy Ridenour is a research assistant at Alberta Hospital Edmonton.

Anne Rochet is an associate professor in the Department of Speech Pathology and Audiology at the University of Alberta in Edmonton.

Akio Tani is a system programmer and analyst at Alberta Hospital Edmonton.

William G. Webster is a professor of psychology and Dean of Social Sciences at Brock University, St. Catherines, Ontario.

Lorne T. Yeudall was the director of the Department of Neuropsychology at Alberta Hospital Edmonton and is currently living in Vancouver and writing a book on Brain and Behavior.

Catherine A. Mateer

1 Neural Bases of Language
Implications for Theories of Stuttering

In the search for working models of stuttering, the clinician/researcher is inevitably drawn to the complex contemporary research on brain/behavior relationships and brain development. In the past decade a wealth of new information, new techniques and new theories have emerged in the neuroscience field that may bear on the complex and fascinating phenomenon we call stuttering. In this paper, brain development, particularly as it relates to cerebral asymmetries—how they come about, what influences them, and what role they may play—is explained. Neural bases of language organization, including both the typical organization in the cortex of motor, sensory and linguistic processes and the patterns which emerge in individuals who demonstrate atypical language lateralization is also focussed on. Finally, the potential relationships between these phenomena and the research on dysfluency are discussed.

Cerebral Asymmetry and Stuttering

Some of the earliest propositions about stuttering to emerge in this century focused on mechanisms of hemisphere interaction. Notions introduced by S.T. Orton (1928) and L.E. Travis (1931) focused on incomplete lateralization of language, competition for language and/or interference effects between hemispheric functioning as pos-

1

sible underpinnings of stuttering behavior. These ideas all refer back in some way to concepts of dominance or relative dominance.

Over the succeeding decades some support for anomalous dominance, including mixed (bilateral) or right hemisphere dominance for speech and language in stutterers has emerged. This has included both behavioral and physiological/anatomical data. The literature on handedness, a factor known to be related, though in no simple way, to cerebral dominance, has fairly consistently reported a higher incidence of left handedness or ambidexterity in the population of individuals who stutter or have other developmental language disorders (Bryngelson and Rutherford, 1937; Geschwind and Behan, 1982). Left-handed individuals have also tended to show a higher incidence of right or mixed cerebral dominance for speech (Milner, Branch and Rasmussen, 1966). There is also at least anecdotal reporting of changes in stuttering behavior when there has been an enforced shift of handedness. In dichotic listening studies, stutterers, as a group, have tended more often to demonstrate a lack of ear preference or an anomalous left ear/right hemisphere advantage for verbal material, suggesting again a mixed or right learning pattern of cerebral organization for language (Rosenfield, 1980).

Alterations in more typical or expected patterns of brain electrical activity, cerebral blood flow, and anatomical asymmetries have also been identified in the stuttering population. Individuals who stutter have demonstrated decreased alpha activity, an indicator of cerebral activation, in the right hemisphere during language processing tasks, whereas nonstutterers usually demonstrate this pattern in the left hemisphere (Moore, Craven and Faber, 1982). In a similar vein, cerebral blood flow, another indicator of cerebral activation, was shown to be increased in the area homologous to Broca's area, but on the right side of the brain, during stuttered speech, but not normally articulated speech. Finally, reversals in or absence of the typical anatomical cerebral asymmetrics have been documented in some, though not all, individuals who stutter.

Despite such reports, which tend to support the notion of atypical cerebral organization in stutterers, much of this research has not been replicated, and conflicting data have been published. Many dichotic listening studies, for example, have demonstrated no clear differences or only very small differences between stutterers and nonstutterers. Handedness surveys and assessments have revealed not only a higher incidence of *strong left* handedness among stutterers but a higher incidence of *strong right* handedness. No study has found differences between all stutterers and all nonstutterers and a number of studies have failed to find any lateralized marker separating any individual stutterer from any individual nonstutterer. The fact that many studies have identified a small group of stutterers who are substantially different in some aspect would appear to argue strongly that stutterers comprise a nonhomogenous population.

The Development of Cerebral Asymmetries

What Is Asymmetrically Represented and When?

Most of the early developmental theorists believed that there was a development of lateralization usually between the age of two and puberty. This belief encompassed the notion that prior to that time there was an equipotentiality between the cerebral hemispheres, such that either hemisphere could subserve language function and development. Included in this camp were Paul Broca, Samuel Orton and Eric Lenneberg.

Since the mid 1970s there has emerged increasing evidence of functional asymmetries in young infants, neonates and even fetuses. Behavioral evidence includes definite head turning and hand use preferences prior to age of one year. It also includes powerful lesion data (Dennis and Whitaker, 1976) which indicates clearly that the hemispheres are not equipotential at an early age. After early lateralized left injury, for example, children show measurable losses in the ability to develop grammatical and syntactic function. Electrophysiological data reported in D.L. Molfese, R.B. Freeman and D.S. Palermo (1975) has indicated left hemisphere specialization for the reception of articulatory patterns and for the kind of rapid acoustic changes that underlie speech perception.

In the past decade, new techniques for brain imaging and cutting have revealed a number of fairly reliable anatomical asymmetries involving the cerebrum. A focus of these studies has been the planum temporale, a region on the superior surface of the temporal lobe that encompasses Broca's area, the center involved in primary speech motor control. This area is larger on the left side of the brain not only in adult, but in infant and fetal brains (Geschwind and Levitsky, 1968; Witelson, 1977). This argues for an innate biologically determined asymmetry from the earliest stages of brain development. Broca's area is actually smaller on the left than the right; this may seem anomalous but is believed to reflect the increased fissuration of the cortex present in the left Broca's area. A third major asymmetry, that of a wider, more protruding frontal pole in the right hemisphere and a wider, more protruding posterior brain volume on the left hemisphere is also seen in adults, children, fetal brains and prehistoric skulls. Such data suggests that the morphological asymmetries in the adult are evident from embryology and are not dependent on experience. According to development biologists, morphologists, and neuroembryologists, patterns of embryological development are ultimately responsible for the structure and form of the adult organism, including the brain, at both gross morphological and histological levels.

Researchers have gradually shifted from simply documenting such asymmetries to asking questions about what they mean and why they have emerged. One possibility is that of a lateralized gradient in maturation. Broca had proposed a left to right maturational shift on purely theoretical grounds. Recent data, however, support a right to left gradient in the embryological emergence and postnatal maturation of the hemispheres. Cortical fissures, for example, consistently appear earlier in the right than in the left fetal hemisphere (Dooling, Chi and Gilles, 1983).

Developmental Gradients and the Emergence of Cerebral Asymmetries

Structural aspects of brain development are complete by an early age. By nine months gestation all cortical and subcortical structures are present. By three years of age, neuron and glial cell counts are fixed and myelinization is 90% that of adult levels. While the subcortex is myelinated by three years of age, myelinization of intracortical cells continues up to 60 years of age. In the study of cerebral lateralization, the structures which serve to interconnect the two massive cerebral hemispheres take on importance. The largest of these communicating fiber bundles is the corpus callosum. New callosal fibers (individual communicating neurons) do not emerge after an early postnatal period. Rather, further development appears to be associated with elimination of fibers. Myelinization of the fibers begins at the end of the fetal period, increases in childhood and plateaus by seven to ten years. Some of these fibers may provide excitation of areas in the opposite hemisphere, some inhibition. The overall growth in size of the callosum, comprised of fibers and myelin is rapid during gestation, low and constant in infancy, and slow after two years on through mid-childhood. While there does not appear to be a sex difference in adult callosal size, once brain weight is taken into account, there may be an interaction between callosal size, sex, and developmental stage.

Recent studies outlined by Catherine Best (1988) have argued for a pattern of fetal brain maturation and growth that takes place in three dimensional space. The three gradients involve the following planes of development:

Right to left

Anterior to posterior

Inferior to superior

The effect of the growth vectors is a counter-clockwise torque evident in the shape of both the developing and the mature brain. The vectors twist the brain forward and ventral on the right and backward and dorsal on the left. This growth pattern is consistent with the major differences in the configuration of the Rolandic and Sylvian fissures and with the earlier appearance of cortical fissuring on the right in the fetus. The only exception to these general patterns is a superimposed fourth growth vector which moves from Primary to Tertiary areas in each of the major brain lobes and is related to the major cortical sensory and motor areas. This results in the forward extension of the prefrontal regions being the last to develop.

What effect does this action have on neuronal organization? Before considering this, one final factor needs to be considered—the development of the six cortical layers. The deepest three layers (layers 6, 5, and 4) project as long myelinated afferent fibers and form the subcor-

tical white matter. Myelination of these fibers results in greater width
and volume. Therefore, if one area has a propensity to develop earlier
there will likely be denser deep cortical layers. Layer 3 (which
includes cell bodies for neurons of the corpus callosum) and layer 2
(which comprises local cortico-cortico connections) are the latest to
develop. These layers contribute substantially to grey matter and to
cortical fissuring. So, the later the development of a cortical area, the
greater the grey to white matter ratio and the greater the amount of
fissuration. Absolute volume, however, may be less. This phenomena
can be seen in Figure 1.1 that demonstrates that the left Broca's area is
smaller but more densely fissured than the right Broca's area homo-
logue. A secondary effect, seen in Figure 1.2 is increased arborization
in this area. In combination, these factors allow increased local intracortical organization. These conditions are found in the left motor,
premotor and primary sensory areas.

There is also neurophysiological evidence that the human cerebral
hemispheres develop at different rates and ages. R.W. Thatcher, R.A.
Walker and S. Giudice (1987) conducted electrophysiological measures of individuals from age two to adulthood. Thatcher used EEG
measures of coherence and phase relation as indirect measures of
cerebral development and organization. He reported two age-depen-
dent categories of change, one a continuous growth vector and one
involving a series of growth spurts. Continuous growth over the age
span was superimposed on an early right, then left hemisphere lead.
The discrete growth spurts appeared at specific anatomical locations
at specific post-natal periods. Frontal regions, for example, demonstrated major coherence shifts early in the right, then left, then right
frontal regions. Thatcher postulates a proliferation of possible connections, then a dying back of connections over the course of development. He further postulates that the timing of these growth spurts
overlaps with the major Piagetian stages or other developmental
milestones.

Overall, these data support an ontogenetic hypothesis of human
cortical development in which there is a genetically programmed
unfolding of specific cortical connections at relatively specific post-
natal stages. Cognitive and perceptual functions may mature devel-

Figure 1.1   Schematic illustrating the smaller yet more fissurated pre-
motor area in the left (*upper*) as compared to the right (*lower*) hemisphere.
This is the most common pattern in adult right-handed individuals. (From
Best, 1988.)

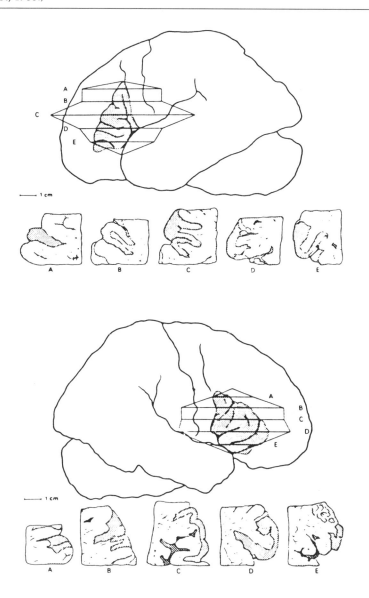

Figure 1.2 Schematic illustrating the greater dendritic arborization in the left than the right pre-motor region. This reflects shorter primary dendritic segments with denser branching and thus more synaptic potential in the left Broca's area. This phenomenon may be dependent on later development of the left anterior cortical region. (From Best, 1988.)

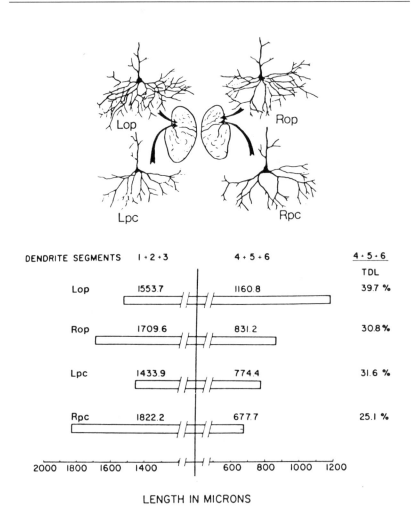

DENDRITE SEGMENTS

	1 + 2 + 3	4 + 5 + 6	4 · 5 · 6
			TDL
Lop	1553.7	1160.8	39.7 %
Rop	1709.6	831.2	30.8 %
Lpc	1433.9	774.4	31.6 %
Rpc	1822.2	677.7	25.1 %

2000 1800 1600 1400   600 800 1000 1200

LENGTH IN MICRONS

opmentally at different rates but within the context of a neural substrata already specialized from the start. Full development of the substrata certainly depends, however, on appropriate external stimulation and exposure. In addition modulation and control of these lateralized gradients of functional maturation and vectors of growth appear to be dependent on both genetic and hormonal factors.

Genetic and Hormonal Factors Influence the Emergence of Cerebral Asymmetries

Some language development disorders, including stuttering, appear to have a clear genetic component. There are also studies which have suggested that, at least in cases of apparently inherited or genetically determined dyslexia, there are alterations in the typical anatomical profile. Rather than demonstrating the expected asymmetry in the planum temporale, these structures tend to be symmetric in dyslexic individuals (Galaburda, Sherman, Rosen, Aboitiz and Geschwind, 1985). There have also been reported microscopic abnormalities in the left perisylvian region (Galaburda, Rosen, Sherman and Assel, 1986). These differences have suggested a disturbance of early neuronal migration. The inference here is that genetic factors affect the growth vector responsible for development in these regions.

There are also reasons to believe that hormonal factors, perhaps under genetic control, have a strong biochemical influence on prenatal neuronal migration and connectivity. Sex hormones have recently come under specific interest. Sex differences in functional brain organization may be mediated by sex differences in maturation rate dependent on fetal hormones. Testosterone, particularly, has been postulated to underlie the increased incidence of learning disability in males and left handers (Geschwind and Behan, 1984). It may play a similar role in some individuals who stutter. As a result of a hormonally based alteration in brain development, the environmental stimulation for speech development may be out of phase with a biologically based maturational timetable.

How might such developmental variation relate to the right to left maturational gradient, including the fact that there appears to be greater plasticity inherent in the later maturation of the left frontal motor and premotor regions? Children comprehend and produce the emotional, intonational and prosodic aspects of speech, features which have been related to right hemisphere function, earlier than they demonstrate comprehension or propositional use of words and word combinations thought to be more left hemisphere dependent tasks (Lewis, 1936). Efficient use of the latter may be dependent on the later maturation of the left hemisphere systems and their capacity for precise and complex cortically based motor control, including that for articulation. Individuals who stutter often do not have difficulty with highly intoned speech or with oral production and articulation during singing. There may have been some limitation in the development of the left hemisphere systems that subserve propositional speech, as a result of hormonal influences on the staging of cerebral maturation.

Emerging data support some degree of normal developmental invariance, yet the timeless constancy of cerebral asymmetries coexists with continuous developmental change on many levels. The child's perceptual, cognitive, motor and linguistic skills change. Neuronal plasticity undergoes developmental change. And the cerebral hemispheres are undergoing continuous charge—in dendriticarborization, in neuronal connectivity, in neurotransmitter function, and in myelinization. Change and constancy are codeterminants of developmental growth in a biological system. Structural and functional properties of the two cerebral hemispheres do change developmentally, but in the context of an ever-present continuous lateral gradient of neuronal differentiation and maturation.

Cerebral Organization for Speech and Language

The phenomenon of stuttering, although primarily a motor output problem affecting fluent articulation, does appear to be closely tied with language and linguistic skill. Stutterers, as a group, tend to demonstrate a somewhat delayed development of language. Stuttering also varies with the degree and propositionality of language, in much the same way that aphasic responses often vary in terms of this factor. Stutterers also do more poorly on a variety of language tasks, including word associations and measures of "sound mindedness" or phonemic analysis. M.E. Wingate (1988) articulates a psycholinguistic view of stuttering based on such observations. Language, in most right-handed individuals is organized in the left cortex. This organization appears, however to be influenced by genetic factors, hormonal factors, developmental factors, gender, brain integrity and experience.

What can the Wada procedure tell us about cerebral asymmetry for speech and language? Some of the research cited earlier has suggested higher incidence of bilateral speech representation or mixed dominance in populations of individuals who stutter. By far the most reliable way of determining cerebral dominance for speech and language is the intracarotid sodiumamytal procedure, first described by J. Wada (1949; Wada and Rasmussen, 1960). In this procedure, a short acting barbiturate is injected into the carotid artery of each hemisphere separately, temporarily shutting down most of the functions of that hemisphere for a period of minutes. In that time, language and memory can be tested to determine the relative dependence of these functions on each hemisphere.

R.K. Jones, in 1966, was the first to report on the language dominance of four individuals who stuttered using intracarotid amytal injections. Each subject demonstrated bilateral representation of language. All four were left handed and each had left handedness in the family. To date there have been 11 studies of individuals who stutter using the Wada technique. Of these only five showed clear support of bilateral speech, while the others did not. This could be interpreted as further support for the nonhomogeneity of stuttering.

Aside from its use in explicating the nature of language dominance in stutterers themselves, the Wada technique has the potential to increase our understanding of the nature of typical and atypical language dominance in a general sense. I had the opportunity to conduct a retrospective analysis of individuals who demonstrated atypical, that is, right or bilateral language dominance on the Wada procedure (Mateer and Dodrill, 1983). There is little information as to the neuropsychological or linguistic status of individuals with verified atypical language organization. We wondered whether language, memory, and other cognitive functions developed to the same extent as in individuals with more typical left hemisphere lateralization. We also asked whether all facets of language were duplicated in each hemisphere of the individuals with bilateral speech or whether some features were shared and others remained the primary province of one hemisphere.

Neuropsychological status, medical history and videotapes made during the amytal procedure were reviewed for 99 subjects. Of that group only 15 were judged to have atypical language lateralization (LL Group), 9 to have evidence of right hemisphere speech representation (RL Group), and 6 to have bilateral speech representation (BL Group). All had a history of seizure disorder. Groups did not differ in age, education or distribution of gender. They did differ on the variable of handedness. While only 19 percent of individuals with typical left hemisphere dominance were left handed, 89 percent of individuals with right hemisphere speech representation and 33 percent of individuals with bilateral speech representation were left handed.

Since these subjects had clear neurological abnormality as indicated by the seizure disorder, we asked whether evidence of early injury might reveal possible reasons for language shift. Although the groups did not differ in their age at seizure onset (overall mean 8.9 years), early history variables were significant.

Only in some cases do seizures appear at all near the time of actual brain injury. It is possible, however, to separate a group of patients in whom early injury, which was presumably etiological to the seizure disorder, was indicated based on the emergence of seizures at a very early age or early documented neurological damage. Using these two criteria, 44 of the 90 patients in this study (49%) demonstrated a positive neurological history prior to the age of seven. In 35 of the 75 patients in the LL group (47%) there was evidence for early damage or dysfunction. In only eight of these 35 was there a strong suggestion based either on etiologic or behavioral variables that the early damage was lateralized. In six, the damage appeared to be related to the right hemisphere, in the remaining two to damage in anterior frontal or temporal regions of the left hemisphere.

There was evidence for early injury in seven of the nine patients in the RL group (78%). Two had porencephalic cysts in the region of the left sensori-motor cortex; two sustained cerebrovascular accidents involving the left middle cerebral artery territory within the first eight months of life, two had the previously mentioned AVM's in the left parietal region and one an episode of meningitis at four and one-half years of age. The first six of these cases demonstrate lateralized damage involving central regions of the left cortex normally considered important to speech and language functions. All of these patients were also left handed. In the case with meningitis, damage is likely to have been more diffuse, or at least nonlateralized; this patient was right handed.

In four of the six BL patients (67%) there was evidence of early damage, but in none of the cases were the effects likely to have been strictly lateralized. In two cases there was documentation of significant perinatal distress or difficulty without lateralizing signs, in one case a suggestion of mild rubella and in another documentation of mushroom poisoning at less than one year of age. Another interesting aspect of the overall analysis was that as adults these subjects as a group demonstrated significant linguistic deficits on an aphasia screening battery.

Overall there was a significantly higher proportion of patients in both the RL and BL groups than in the LL Group who demonstrated evidence of neurological damage before the age of seven. In six of the seven RL patients with early damage the affected area(s) included central regions of the left cortex which are normally considered important to speech and language functions. This finding is in keeping with data from Rasmussen and Milner (1977) suggesting that early damage to speech regions can result in a switch to dependence on right hemisphere systems. Of those patients in the BL group with early damage (4/6), the damage appeared in all cases to have been diffuse. Patients in the LL group appeared to have the lowest incidence of early neurological injury, and when it occurred it was more likely to have been nonlateralized, or in the right hemisphere. When lateralized to the left hemisphere (n=2) it did not involve central left cortical areas commonly related to language functions. In those LL cases, perhaps, there was no reason to develop language outside of typical "language areas."

We next asked whether all aspects of speech and language were represented on the "dominant" side and whether in the cases of bilateral speech, certain speech functions were dually or separately represented in each hemisphere. To answer this a detailed linguistic analysis of speech errors made during the amytal perfusions of each hemisphere was carried out (Mateer and Dodrill, 1983). Responses on a sentence reading task were analyzed for four types of errors: phonemic/articulatory errors, grammatic/syntactic errors, semantic errors and jargon. Results are given in Table 1.1. The LL group clearly showed a greater preponderance of all error types with the left hemisphere perfusion. The RL group demonstrated a significantly greater number of phonemic/articulatory, grammatic/syntactic and jargon errors after the right-sided than the left-sided perfusion, although only jargon errors reached significance. Semantic errors were more equally represented following perfusion of either side. Within the BL group, no significant differences between the left and right perfusion on the incidence of any error type was found. Yet, there was a strong tendency for phonemic/articulatory errors and grammatic/syntactic errors to occur more frequently with left as opposed to right sided injection. Thus, even when speech is bilaterally represented the usual pre-eminence of the left hemisphere for sequencing, which is involved in articulation and syntactic structuring, emerges. Only when speech is clearly shifted to the right are articulatory functions carried out by that hemisphere. Semantic aspects of language appeared to be represented to a similar degree in both hemispheres in the right dominant and bilateral language groups.

Intrahemispheric Organization of Speech and Language

A large body of data regarding the intrahemispheric organization of language in the left cortical and subcortical structures has emerged from the aphasiology literature. Although many aphasic patients

Table 1.1   Means and standard deviations of errors on the sentence reading task by linguistic type and side of perfusion for individuals with left, right, and bilateral language representation

Reading error type	Language lateralization		
	Left (LL) (n = 9)	Right (RL) (n = 9)	Bilateral (BL) (n = 6)
Phonemic/articulatory			
Left perfusion	2.7 (2.5)	0.9 (1.1)	1.3 (1.6)
Right perfusion	0.9 (1.5)[a]	1.7 (2.1)	0.2 (0.4)
Grammatic/syntactic			
Left perfusion	2.6 (2.6)	0.7 (0.8)	4.7 (4.1)
Right perfusion	0.7 (1.1)[a]	2.3 (3.7)	2.3 (3.4)
Semantic			
Left perfusion	2.7 (1.9)	2.1 (1.8)	1.8 (1.7)
Right perfusion	0.9 (1.5)[a]	1.5 (1.6)	2.0 (1.1)
Jargon			
Left perfusion	1.6 (1.6)	0.0	0.7 (1.6)
Right perfusion	0.0[a]	2.7 (3.6)[a]	1.7 (2.7)

[a] $p < 0.01$ (intragroup left/right perfusion effects)

have large lesions which disrupt many aspects of both expressive and receptive language, a few aphasias are characterized by restricted linguistic disruption. These could be considered to include the agrammatic, anomic, and conduction aphasias. These are usually the result of smaller lesions not directly involving the perisylvian cortex. Persistent aphasia usually involves large portions of the perisylvian cortex and/or its underlying connections. Overall fluency of speech output usually decreases as there is encroachment on the anterior perisylvian motor and premotor regions (Mateer, 1989).

I had the opportunity to conduct a finer grained analysis of cortical sites involved in speech and language in the course of conducting a large number of intraoperative cortical mapping procedures with individuals undergoing neurosurgical procedures. Responses to sentence reading, naming, oral movement sequencing trials, and phonemic identification tasks were analyzed during electrical stimulation of cortical sites (Mateer, 1983; Ojemann and Mateer, 1979). Stimulation of the dominant cortex during the reading of simple sentences has demonstrated unexpected patterns of linguistic alteration. The major error categories associated with stimulation-related alteration include speech arrest (an inability to produce any speech), articulatory (phonetic or phonemic) errors, grammatic errors, and semantic errors.

Articulatory errors were divided into literal paraphasias (productions that displayed acceptable phonological form but contained less than 50 percent of the phones of the target word; i.e., "If next winzer is worth and sucks. . . ."). Sites associated with articulatory/phonological errors were distributed broadly but always within the perisylvian cortex.

Grammatic errors associated with stimulation were widely distributed throughout superior temporal, parietal, and frontal regions of the left lateral cortex. Disruptions of grammar with stimulation of sites in the mid-superior temporal lobe and parietotemporal region were similar to the paragrammatic deficit seen in aphasic patients with posterior lesions. These aphasic patients often misuse function words and demonstrate errors in verb forms, though all parts of grammar are represented. An example of a grammatic error made during electrical stimulation of the posterior temporal lobe is "She will be visit the mountain."

Semantic errors were, like grammatic errors, distributed widely in frontal, temporal, and parietal regions. Semantic errors include productions marked by inappropriate meaning (e.g., "Should the soup be too salty, you can add in salt water"), as well as productions marked by categorical substitutions (soldier/sailor, mother/sister). Overall the pattern of cortical organization revealed in this analysis suggested that the motoric execution of speech as reflected in speech sound selection and production (articulatory/phonological errors)

Figure 1.3   Linguistic alterations during reading associated with cortical stimulation. Sites statistically associated with a single type of linguistic change when stimulation was applied during a reading task are shown. Sites marked by diamonds were associated only with articulatory/phonological errors and cluster in the perisylvian core. These sites are also associated with sequencing of oral movements and phonemic perception. Sites marked by triangles and stars mark sites associated with grammatic and semantic errors, respectively. They tend to be broadly distributed but are generally located at least one gyrus distal to the sylvian fissure.

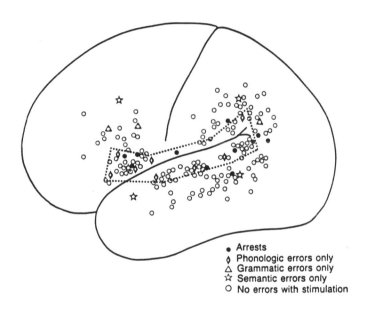

was highly dependent on the perisylvian core. Both the traditional anterior "motor" area and the posterior perisylvian areas were critically involved. Aspects of reading relating to more linguistically based aspects of language, including grammatic and semantic selection, occupy more distal sites. The concentric "ring-like" appearance of the distributions (Figure 1.3) is highly reminiscent of the concentric field features associated with the primary, secondary, and tertiary association fields of other major cortical motor and sensory systems.

Insight into motor mechanisms supporting speech/language function was obtained by mapping the effects of cortical stimulation on the ability to mimic repeated single and sequential orofacial movements (Mateer, 1983; Ojemann and Mateer, 1979). These studies were prompted by the observations of Mateer and Kimura (1977) that the ability to mimic sequential facial movements is altered in both fluent and nonfluent aphasic patients compared to either normal subjects or those with brain damage not associated with aphasia. Repetition of the same movement was disrupted with stimulation of sites only in face pre-motor cortex. This region corresponds roughly to, but is smaller than, the traditional motor speech area. In all cases, these sites were also associated with arrests on naming and reading suggesting that these sites represent part of the cortical pathway for orofacial movement that is critical for speech. It is not part of the face motor cortex per se, as oral or facial movements were not evoked. Sequences of oral movements were disrupted over a broader area from sites throughout the extent of perisylvian cortex and well outside the classic sensorimotor cortex.

Disruption of consonant identification was also evoked from a broad range of perisylvian cortex. Of interest was the high degree of overlap between sites associated with disrupted phoneme identification and disrupted sequencing of oral movements. These changes localized a region in language cortex important for oral motor sequencing and phonemic identification, functions critically involved in speech production and comprehension. It was hypothesized that these areas of perisylvian cortex, involved in both the production of oral movement sequences and the perception of phonemes, provide the neural substrate for much of the basic production and perception of speech. This perisylvian region is clearly implicated when one looks at sites that altered articulatory/phonological aspects on the reading task. The extent of lesions that give rise to a permanent motor aphasia, as identified by Mohr (1976), also encompasses this same perisylvian region. This area is crucial for the generation of language, and damage to it is hypothesized to account for phonemically based production and comprehension deficits associated with most aphasias. Many of these production errors may include those errors sometimes incorporated under the term *verbal apraxia*.

How might we relate this new perspective on the close integration of speech production and perception to stuttering? Stuttering reflects at some level and for whatever reason a diminished capacity to select, coordinate, and produce motor acts under the influence of sensory feedback. Rosenfield and Nudelman (1987) postulate that individuals who stutter have a brain at risk for developing problems with speech output, that their speech motor control systems are closer to an "instability threshold." These individuals may lack the capacity to deal with the relationship between motor acts and associated sensory stimuli resulting in a decreased capability of generating fine temporal programs for the integration of input and output. Given unreliability in such a system, it would make sense that the peak onset of stuttering is at a time when explosive growth in language capacity outstrips an immature or undeveloped speech motor control apparatus and that the peak age for recovery should be when motor abilities catch up with language demands. It also makes sense that fluency evoking measures such as slowed speech and air flow regulation work because they decrease the frequency or speed of the stuttering movements and thus increase stability. Of course, we have focused here primarily on evidence from cortical stimulation studies, which addressed the role of cortical structures in speech motor control. Many other parts of the brain are involved in oral motor control including the cerebellum, the basal ganglia, the thalamus and the supplementary motor cortex (SMA). William Webster later in this volume articulates a theory of stuttering which focuses on dysfunction of the SMA and its role in regulation of interhemispheric communication (Webster, 1988).

Gender Differences and the Role of Sex Hormones

In the course of cortical mapping studies, a substantial degree of variability was seen in the cortical organization of language from person to person. Some of this variability appeared to relate to gender differences. Evoked changes in naming were evoked from a smaller area of the left cortex in females than in males. Males appeared, in particular, to be more dependent on posterior parietal regions for naming than did women (Mateer, Polen, and Ojemann, 1982). This is consistent with other data reported by Kimura (1980) in which she describes sex differences in intrahemispheric organization of speech in patients with acquired vascular lesions. Thus sex hormones appear to play a role, not only in patterns of interhemispheric development, but in intrahemispheric organization as well. Motor programming critical for speech and manual activity is not only just as lateralized in females, it also appears more focally organized in the left anterior regions. The superior manual dexterity and speech fluency of females may be related to this more focal organization in left motor regions. There is also new data suggesting that levels of sex hormone can influence abilities in the adult. Hormonal influences appear to be selective, increasing some skills while decreasing others. Kimura (1989) reported that when estrogen and progesterone levels are high in female humans, there is a decline in performance on visual perceptual tasks and an increase in speeded manual movement and articulation tasks. A similar enhancement has been reported during the estrogen phase of hormone replacement in menopausal women.

It is possible then, that regions of the left hemisphere may prove to be among the brain areas sensitive to the activational effects of sex hormones. It appears that the hormonal environment may modify cognitive patterns within the limits of genetic predisposition. The higher incidence of male stutterers may relate in some way to this phenomenon.

What Is Gained from Reports of Acquired Dysfluency?

The literature is now replete with references to acquired dysfluency or stuttering. Yet little evidence has emerged from this literature to assist with a theory of stuttering or its cause. Usually the dysfluencies and associated speech/language deficits are poorly described. Acquired neurologically based stuttering has been reported following both right and left hemisphere lesions, following unilateral and bilateral lesions, following anterior and posterior lesions, and subcortical as well as cortical lesions. The lack of objective neurological data in most stutterers would argue strongly against any particular site of lesion. In addition, acquired stuttering usually does not have all the characteristics of developmental stuttering and so may be quite different in origin. What the literature does, however, is reveal the extent of cortical control that is required for effective speech output, and reinforce the concept of stuttering as a symptom which can result from disruption of a variety of neurologic systems.

The Challenge

How can we relate any of the new and exciting information emerging to the phenomenon of stuttering? All stutterers would seem to have a disruption in the mechanism for speech motor control. Some may have a disturbance in laterality resulting from genetic, hormonal, or other factors which influence developmental growth factors in fetal life or infancy. These vectors and stages of growth appear to critically influence the patterns of cerebral asymmetries and cortical development that lay the groundwork for adult behavior.

This review suggested some of the critical developmental sequences which may be necessary to assure specialized neuronal circuitry in the left motor and premotor regions. These regions were later seen to be critical in the speech production/speech perception interface. Since so many systems need to be coordinated, over time and in the context of developmental, genetic, hormonal, and environmental factors, stuttering might emerge from a variety of sources or mechanisms, consistent with the heterogeneity that is seen in the research on this population. In addition, stuttering is not only developed in, but appears to be maintained by social context and emotional factors.

Neuroscience often leaves us with conflicting findings from different methodologies. Yet the enormous complexity of the brain, its organization, and its development argues against simplistic or singular explanations for any behavior as complex as speech. New developments in neuroscience and neurolinguistics may, however, lead us to ask more probing and effective questions which will lead us to a better understanding of dysfluency, its origins and its treatment.

References

Best, C.T. (1988). The emergence of cerebral asymmetries in early human development: A literature review and a neuroembryological model. In D.L. Molfese and S.T. Segalowitz, eds., *Brain lateralization in children: Developmental implications.* New York: Guilford Press.

Bryngelson, B. and Rutherford, B. (1937). A comparative study of laterality of stutterers and non-stutterers. *Journal of Speech Disorders* 2: 15–16.

Dennis, M. and Whitaker, H.A (1976). Language acquisition following hemidecortication: Linguistic superiority of the left over right hemisphere. *Brain and Language* 9: 206–14.

Dooling, E.C., Chi, J.G., and Gilles, G.H. (1983). Telencephalic development: Changing gyral patterns. In F.H. Gilles, A. Leviston and E.C. Dooling, eds., *The developing human brain: Growth and epidemiologic neuropathy,* pp. 94–104. Boston: John Wright, PSG.

Galaburda, A.M., Rosen, G.D., Sherman, G.F. and Assel, E. (1986). Neuropathological findings in a woman with developmental dyslexia. *Annals of Neurology* 20: 170.

Galaburda, A.M., Sherman, G.F., Rosen, G.D., Aboitiz, F. and Geschwind, N. (1985). Developmental dyslexia: Four consecutive patients with cortical anomalies. *Annals of Neurology* 18: 222–33.

Geschwind, N. and Behan, P.U. (1982). Left-handedness: Association with immune disease, migraine and developmental learning disorders. *Proceedings at the National Academy of Sciences* 79: 5057–5100.

———. (1984). Laterality, hormones and immunity. In N. Geschwind and A.M. Galaburda, eds., *Cerebral dominance: The biological foundations,* pp. 211–24. Cambridge, MA: Harvard University Press.

Geschwind, N. and Levitsky, W. (1968). Human brain: Left-right asymmetries in temporal speech region. *Science* 161: 186.

Jones, R.K. (1966). Observations on stammering after localized cerebral injury. *Journal of Neurology, Neurosurgery and Psychiatry* 27: 142–45.

Kimura, D. (1980). Sex differences in intrahemispheric organization of speech. *Behavioral and Brain Sciences* 3: 215–63.

Lewis, M.M. (1936). *Infant speech: A study of the beginnings of language.* New York: Academic Press.

Mateer, C. (1983). Localization of language and visuospatial functions by electrical stimulation. In H. Whitaker, ed., *Localization in neuropsychology.* New York: Academic Press.

———. (1989). Neural correlates of language function. In D.P. Kuehn, M.L.

Lemne and J.M. Baumgartner, eds., *Neural bases of speech, hearing, and language*. Boston: College-Hill Press.

Mateer C. and Dodrill, C. (1983). Neuropsychological and linguistic correlates of atypical language lateralization: Evidence from sodium amytal studies. *Human Neurobiology* 2: 135–42.

Mateer, C., Polen S., and Ojemann, G.A. (1982). Sexual variation in cortical localization of naming as determined by stimulation mapping. *Behavioral and Brain Sciences* 5: 310–11.

Milner, B., Branch, C. and Rasmussen, T. (1966). Evidence for bilateral speech representation in some non-right-handers. *Trans. American Neurological Association* 91: 306–8.

Mohr, J. (1976). Broca's area and Broca's aphasia. *Studies in Neurolinguistics* 1: 201–36.

Molfese, D.L., Freeman, R.B. and Palermo, D.S. (1975). The ontogeny of brain lateralization for speech and nonspeech stimuli. *Brain and Language* 2: 356–68.

Moore, W.H., Jr., Craven, D.C. and Faber, M.M. (1982). Hemispheric alpha asymmetries of words with positive, negative and neutral arousal values preceding tasks of recall and recognition: Electrophysiological and behavioral results from stuttering males and nonstuttering males and females. *Brain and Language* 19: 211–24.

Ojemann, G.A. and Mateer, C. (1979). Human language cortex: localization of memory, syntax and segvertial motor-phoneme identification systems. *Science* 205: 1401–3.

Orton, S.T. (1928) A physiological theory of reading disability and stuttering in children. *New England Journal of Medicine* 198: 1045–52

Rasmussen, T. and Milner B. (1977). The role of early left brain injury in determining lateralization of cerebral speech function. *Annals of the New York Academy of Science* 299: 355–69.

Rosenfield, D.R. (1980). Cerebral dominance and stuttering. *Journal of Fluency Disorders* 5: 171–85.

Rosenfield, D.R., and Nudelman, H.B. (1987). Neuropsychological models of speech dysfluency. In L. Rustin, H. Purser and D. Rowley, eds., *Progress in the treatment of fluency disorders*. London: Taylor and Francis.

Thatcher, R.W., Walker, R.A., and Giudice, S. (1987). Human cerebral hemispheres develop at different rates and ages. *Science* 230: 110–13.

Travis, L.E. (1931). *Speech pathology*. New York: Appleton.

Wada, J. (1949). A new method for the determination of the side of cerebral dominance: A preliminary report on the intracarotid injection of sodium amytal in man. *Igaku to Scibutsugaku* (Medicine and Biology) 14: 221–22 (Japanese).

Wada, J. and Rasmussen T. (1960). Intracarotid injection of sodium amytal for the lateralization of cerebral speech dominance. *Journal of Neurosurgery* 17: 266–82.

Webster, W. G. (1988). Neural mechanisms underlying stuttering: Evidence from bimanual handwriting performance. *Brain and Language* 33: 226–44.

Wingate, M. E. (1988). *The structure of stuttering: A psycho-linguistic analysis.* New York: Springer Verlag.

Witelson, S.F. (1977). Early hemisphere specialization and interhemispheric plasticity: An empirical and theoretical review. In S. Segalowitz and F.A. Gruder, eds., *Language development and neurological theory.* New York: Academic Press.

Discussion

H. Gregory: As a first question I want to refer to the review that you gave of the interest in the relationship between laterality and stuttering. Our group wants you to comment on whether the emphasis should be not so much on laterality but rather on the efficiency of certain processing that is related to language, to dysfluency and stuttering.

C. Mateer: I think that is a very good point. I would really concur with the spirit of that although I can certainly be considered a localizationist based on my background. I really feel that functions in the brain are organized discretely in some very consistent, repeatable and reliable ways, that unfold through development. By no means do any parts of the brain or sides of the brain ever function in isolation. Rather, all parts of the brain need to function together in a very coordinated and integrated way. I think that the emphasis on laterality in my opening remarks is really one of relative dominance. There is a balance of power between the hemispheres, a little bit like detente. We should be looking at what is and is not shared across the hemispheres and how that sharing is more or less effective. I was quite struck in looking at individuals under sodium amytal procedures, as I showed earlier, at how much contribution there is from each of the hemispheres, although in somewhat different ways in each of the individuals that we saw. I would concur with reducing the emphasis on laterality, at least in the sense that it conveys dominance, and focusing rather on efficiency and the way in which functions are shared, both across the hemispheres and, very interestingly, within each of the hemispheres.

H. Gregory: Our next question is related to the first. We were very interested in the diagrams that you showed about brain stimulation studies and we saw a lot of overlap in the various language functions that were pictured. We would like you to talk more about the overlap that is related to language and the implications for stuttering.

C. Mateer: When we mapped language functions in the dominant and nondominant hemisphere we did not evoke many language changes in the nondominant right hemisphere so we quickly moved to doing a series of studies related to visual spatial processing. Within the left hemisphere, in addition to looking at object naming, we also looked at the ability to read and to complete sentences. For example, the individual saw a sentence frame. It consisted of a dependent clause followed by an independent clause but the verb form of the independent clause was missing. Thus, for example the patient might see, "If my son is late for class again he," a long blank and then the word "principal." What they would have to do when that slide came on is read the slide and fill in the blank with the appropriate word or words. We designed the blanks so that they would have to generate a grammatically inflected verb form. Then we presented sentences like that on multiple occasions with stimulation at multiple sites. Responses were recorded and we subsequently analyzed the sentence productions for errors and categorized them according to whether they were articulatory errors, grammatical errors, syntactic errors or semantic errors. Then we would determine whether or not a particular site was associated with that kind of error. We threw out any samples where a patient made errors just like they made on nonstimulation trials and focused on errors that were made *only* under conditions of cortical stimulation. We required repeated samples of the same kind of error before we would associate a particular site on the cortex with a particular function. We ended up with a whole set of sites where, on sentence reading, there were clear repeatable disruptions of articulatory functions (e.g., pencil for tencil), or grammatical functions, (e.g., errors involving incorrect inflected verb forms). Sometimes patients made semantic errors, which were really word substitutions, or completions of the sentence with something that did not make any sense from a semantic perspective. When we plotted these out, we ended up with a broad distribution of each error type. Sites were identified in the frontal, temporal and parietal lobes related to articulation. In all cases these were within one gyrus of the parisylvian fissure. We never evoked articulatory errors from sites that were distal from the parisylvian fissure by more than one gyrus. They all clustered quite closely in the parisylvian region. There were many sites where stimulation resulted in arrest of speech in the motor or premotor region on the left side. We could not analyze these sites any further because they just could not say anything. They might just get one syllable out and then stop. When we looked at sites at which stimulation evoked grammatical changes, we found those sites also to be distributed quite widely. However, they tended to be, when isolated, more distal from the parisylvian fissure. When they were near the parisylvian fissure they were always made in conjunction with articulation errors. Semantic errors were always more distal, never in the parisylvian region and never associated with articulation. Next we looked at the oral motor mapping studies and phoneme perception studies.

The model we developed out of these studies includes a primary area in the premotor region on the left cortex where you get disruption of speech, of any kind of articulation or even single movements. There is an area like that on the right but it is much smaller and more discrete. Then there is a surrounding region that is important to the sequencing of movement includ-

ing nonverbal oral movement. It is also important to the selection and sequencing of speech sounds and to the perception of
speech sounds; a kind of central articulatory-motor-perceptual
core in the parisylvian region. More distal to that, and surrounding it, are sites where we get disruption of more linguistically based functions and beyond that another range where
we have disruption of short-term verbal memory. It is almost
like peeling an onion where the core of the onion, the parisylvian cortex, relates to motor sequencing, both verbal and nonverbal and to phoneme perception, with outer layers involving
more linguistic and then memory sites. That kind of organization, we think, fits much better with lesion work than some of
the more traditional notions about an anterior/posterior or
expressive/receptive dichotomy.

H. Gregory: Would you make a brief comment on the blood flow
studies and your feelings about the kind of information that we
can get from them. We were interested in the one study that
you reported where there was stuttering, or no stuttering,
depending on changes in blood flow.

C. Mateer: I do not have the reference on the top of my head about
that study but it intrigued me as well. As I recall it indicated a
nonconstant right hemisphere activation during speech in a
stutterer. The right hemisphere was activated only during a
stuttering act. It would seem to me that if this finding were real
and could be repeated it would be quite interesting. In regard
to blood flow studies generally, it is a relatively new but very
promising technique. Unlike many of the other imaging measures like CT scan and MRI scan, which really only tell us
something about structural integrity, the cerebral blood flow
studies and the PET scan studies tell us something about how
different parts of the brain are functioning during certain
activities.

There are still many problems relating to interpretation of
cerebral blood flow changes. The idea is that an increase in

blood flow is related to an increase in the uptake of nutrients and that implies a higher rate of functioning. That higher level of functioning may reflect a positive or a negative effect in that it may be excitatory or inhibitory. We really do not know, when we get increased activity in a region, exactly what that region is doing. I think it is a very exciting and an interesting new technique and I would like to see it used more.

R. Kroll: Dr. Mateer, our group also appreciated your most stimulating and informative talk and we were intrigued by the concept of subgroups that you mentioned on a number of occasions. Many of us working clinically with stutterers have considered the concept of subgroups time and time again because there are those that do well in therapy and those who react somewhat differently. Our discussion continued on to a discussion of other kinds of disorders such as neurogenic or acquired stuttering, apraxia and cluttering. We wonder if you see these disorders as representing different points on a continuum of speech motor disorders?

C. Mateer: The issue is whether these different kinds of motor control disorders are operating on some kind of continuum. That might imply a clear gradation from one point to another or different nodes of possible disruption in a system of motor control. With regard to apraxia this has certainly been an abiding interest of mine. My studies in oral movement control and oral movement sequencing were basically an attempt to look at the relationship between apraxia, a motor selection and programming sequencing disorder, and aphasia. I have been quite struck with the degree of relationship between the inability to produce single oral movements of the mouth, face, tongue, articulators and the ability to produce single speech sounds. There is also a very high correlation in patients with lesions between difficulty with the selection and sequencing of oral and speech movements. So I see a high degree of relationship between what we think of as

oral apraxia and aphasia. Motor selection disorders may underlie many of the aphasic problems that we see. In that sense I certainly see the motor control system as interrelated with the linguistic system.

I can certainly extend that motor control hypothesis, particularly with its heavy dependence on feedback loops, evident in
strong relationships between production and perception, to the
stuttering literature that I have seen. Some of the data I showed
suggests that rather than thinking about anterior systems as
critically important for speech expression, we also depend, in a
very important way, on posterior temporal and parietal systems for motor control. In a similar fashion we do not just
depend on posterior sensory systems for auditory based phonemic perceptions. If you recall all those little sites marked with
"◊'s" at the front of my diagram [Figure 1.3], you will be
reminded that the anterior regions of the brain, including
Broca's area, are very important for single phoneme perception.
Many patients with Broca's aphasia have a great deal of difficulty not only with expression but also with reception of single
phonemes. I think all of these different disorders are strongly
interrelated. I think they represent nodes of disruption when
aspects of motor sequencing and control systems that support
language are disrupted.

The first of your questions was about subgroups. It seemed
to me, as I was looking through the studies, that it is doubtful
there will be one single reason for dysfluency or stuttering
behavior. Consider the fact that you can get lesions in so many
different places in the brain and acquire the disorder; consider
the fact that there are so many differences even in individuals
with idiopathic stuttering. I do not know what the best break-
downs would be—whether they may be on a genetic basis or
on a hormonal basis. You probably have other ideas of what
would comprise useful groupings.

R. Kroll: Our group talked about how at one point in the history of
our research we addressed neural mechanisms and central pro-

cessing in stuttering. For the next 20–25 years or so we became more involved in studying the peripheral behaviors of stuttering. Would you support, in a research sense, getting away from studying stuttering from a symptomatic or behavioral point of view and spending much more energy and time developing our methodology to study the central processing?

C. *Mateer:* I guess at some level we really have to keep in mind that stuttering is a behavior and we have to look at the behavior and recognize that the behavior does reflect both central and peripheral mechanisms. So I certainly would not suggest that efforts to look at and quantify things like voice onset time, movement parameters, or ways in which structures are coarticulating are inappropriate. Those are the things that we can really measure and they are the behaviors. I think it is certain that these things do not operate independent of a central control mechanism. We need to use those peripheral measurements as a way to quantify the behaviors we are describing and get a better handle on what is happening. We must keep in mind, however, that they have a central substrata and always refer back to what that might be. When I did the video pictures of people sticking out their tongue, it was interesting because it gave us some idea about selection and execution of movement but it really was not enough to quantify things. I went on to studies of voice onset time and to gather more finely detailed aspects of movement control during cortical stimulation. So I think there must be a meld between studies of behavior and inferences about central processing; they cannot be disassociated.

R. *Kroll:* If we look at some of the diagrams in the research that you have presented in terms of representation in the brain and the real scattering of symptoms that you get with various stimulations and if we accept a neurophysiological model of stuttering as being perhaps diffusely located in the brain, might we not also accept concomitant or other deficits in areas such as visual, motor or any of the areas that you may have alluded to?

C. Mateer: I think you are asking whether I would expect to see concomitant changes in stutterers in other aspects of behavior or
cognition. Yes, I think there is no doubt that one would expect
them. I think that if we begin looking and pushing a little bit we
will see evidence emerging that more general linguistic capabilities, more general perceptual capabilities, other associated
movement capabilities related to other systems of the body,
manual movements, and eye movements may also be involved.
We should perhaps not look so focally at stuttering behavior
but look more broadly at things that may be more subtle but
give us good clues as to what parts of the brain or what
processes or functions may be involved.

R. Kroll: Is there any research on brain stimulation for very young
children? One of our concerns was that we are doing a lot of
research on the brains of adult stutterers after they have
acquired behavioral and emotional responses to the stuttering.

C. Mateer: No, not that I know of. The reason for doing these sorts of
cortical mapping studies is certainly not for research, although
it is nice to get some research data as well. These studies are
undertaken for clinical purposes, that is, for the safe resection
of epileptic foci. Other applications might involve a tumor, for
which they do not know what surgical approach to take. We
can use mapping to identify what would be the safest approach.
I have seen a couple of tumors sitting right in Broca's area in
persons who had absolutely no speech deficits. Presumably,
with a slow growing tumor, speech functions are pushed aside
and relocated but you have no idea where they have relocated
to. By mapping around the area you can usually identify these
sites. In fact we identified an area which functioned like Broca's
area sitting right up on top where the arm cortex would usually
be. We also identified one further back in the posterior temporal lobe. The idea is that you can go in for a safer approach to
tumor resection with such knowledge. But these studies would
only be done in an adult. We just do not feel that children are
really capable of going through the rigors of that kind of opera-

tion. When children are operated on it is usually done under general anesthetic and the child is asleep.

The other kinds of approaches that we have talked about, cerebral blood flow, MRI and PET studies, are certainly being done on children. I talked about cortical mapping but there is also subcortical mapping. Stimulation of subcortical structures, including basal ganglia, thalamus and cerebellum, have also been associated with changes in speech behavior. There are many subcortical areas that appear to be involved in language and speech behaviors.

A. Caruso: Our group really found your presentation on the neural basis of language stimulating [this pun intended]. We thought your presentation laid a good ground work for this whole conference and that it was advantageous to have it at the beginning.

We did generate a number of really good questions and I will try to summarize them as best I can. First let me make the comment that someone in the group wanted me to express and then ask a question about a related comment. The stutterers that you cited in the Jones study, were pre-operatively brain damaged. Is that not the case?

C. Mateer: My understanding is that they stuttered and then developed, as an adult, a neurological problem that had to be addressed. I do not know what the underlying neurologic problem was. Does anyone else?

W. Moore: I do. Three of them had subarachnoid bleeds of sudden onset. One had a tumor, a young child about 15 years of age, for six months duration. All had stuttered since childhood.

C. Mateer: So they were all late developing neurological problems. If it was something like a seizure focus it could have had a much more long standing onset but with subarachnoid hemorrhage, probably not.

A. Caruso: A related question about that whole procedure, not necessarily that particular study. What is the evidence that you use for bilateral speech representation? Is it that both left and right injections led to a cessation or disruption of speech or is it that neither injection led to it?

C. Mateer: That is a really interesting question. I looked at this data in a retrospective way because another neuropsychologist had already made the determination about speech dominance. It was always made on the basis of significant disruption of speech following injections of both hemispheres. Usually there was a stoppage of speech or speech arrest for some seconds or minutes following injection. Then there is a clear disruption of language. However, he made the decision based solely on there being disruption of speech with injection of both sides of the brain. Another way to think about that would certainly be to get disruption from either side, with the assumption that the other side was taking over speech function.

There is a real flaw in all the sodium amytal work that is done. The criteria for what determines language, particularly bilateral language, are not at all clear. How much disruption do you have to get from both sides? What do we do if you do not get it from either side? There are no clear answers to these questions. There are many studies where minimal effects are seen because the drug dosage is not large enough. People's vascular systems are variable and you have to differentiate the dosages for larger people or smaller people. So there are studies where you just do not feel you have had a significant effect. It seems to me that if you get disruption from either side, that might suggest that both sides could be functional for language. But I do not know what those people look like because they were thrown out in this particular series and considered invalid studies.

A. Caruso: Relative to the electrical stimulation studies on the left hemisphere that you talked about, would you comment on comparable studies on the right hemisphere?

C. Mateer: With regard to language functions, nondominant hemisphere stimulation is pretty uneventful. You can get an arrest of
speech. Speech is commonly arrested with stimulation of the
motor face cortex on the right and sometimes a little way into
the pre-motor cortex. We have never had any disruption of
articulatory function, semantic, grammatic or syntactic functions from the right cortex, in any of the studies that I have
done. So rather than continuing those studies we went to a
series of spatial studies and looked at the ability to do some
perceptual matching.

Patients had to match an angle of a line. There would be one
line at the top at a certain angle and three below. They would
just have to say "a," "b" or "c," whichever one it matched. Or
they would have to match faces. There would be one face at the
top and three below and they would just have to match the
face. Or they would have to do a spatial manipulation task. We
had a spatial rotation task for which they had to flip designs
around to a different orientation in their head. Then we would
show them three lines and ask them which one they had seen,
or three faces and ask which they had seen. We had one more
task where we showed them facial expressions. They had to tell
us what kind of facial expression it was. Was it happy, sad,
angry or whatever? So we had angle and face matching, angle
and face memory, a perceptual rotation and a judgement of an
emotional expression. They just had to label it. We found that
we got disruption of perceptual matching from a small premotor site and from a parietal site. We got disruptions of memory
for angles or faces from superior temporal sites. We got very
interesting alterations in the way patients labeled the expression of faces from stimulation at middle temporal gyrus sites.
So it looked as though we could differentially disrupt spatial
matching, memory, and judgement of facial expression with
focal right cortical stimulation. These sites never overlapped.
We never had the same kind of error at the same site. They
were always quite discrete. That argues somewhat against not
having a fair degree of specificity and focal organization in the
right hemisphere.

A. Caruso: In your talk you discussed the probabilities of stuttering occurring with different types of communications. That concept seems to overlap with aphasia, with the inference being that stuttering is perhaps related to some more general language function or process. One of the concerns was that a very similar sort of comment could be made with Parkinson's disease, between the symptomatology of Parkinsonian speech and stuttering. The question that we want to ask you is basically this. One member of our group talked about the relationship between stuttering and other types of disorders, be it language or motor control, a kind of proof by analogy. Could you comment on the vulnerability of generating hypotheses, or at least working notions, on that sort of basis.

C. Mateer: I do not feel that I have generated a particular hypothesis about it. In reading through some things it seemed to me that there was the same kind of hierarchy operating across disorders. Automatic speech, swearing, and synchronous speech are much less likely to be stuttered whereas more propositional speech is more likely to be stuttered. It just struck me when looking for some correlates that individuals with left hemisphere lesions show the same kind of propensity. The suggestion is that it is right hemisphere mechanisms that are capable of generating and reeling off these nonpropositional, emotionally toned and more undifferentiated kinds of speech. That is just to explain the analogy. I certainly agree that it is not something on which we can base a theory. It suggests correlation rather than causation. This might be for a variety of different reasons. I think we need to be looking for some commonalities in the system. It is real easy to focus on one particular disorder and see it as very different than anything else. The most striking example of that is focusing on apraxia and saying that this is purely motor and has nothing to do with anything else or this is aphasia and has nothing to do with motor control. In fact this ignores the strong correlation between motor control and linguistic productions. With regard to the issue of Parkinson's disease, I would not be surprised by parallels. Subcortical basal ganglia systems interact closely with the cortical system. I share your concern about not drawing conclusions on that basis but I think it is helpful to cross fertilize between different fields, working with different pieces of the "elephant" of motor control disorders. We may find more similarities and directions for questioning than we would by seeing them as so different.

A. Caruso: There seem to be a number of processes, perhaps language processes, perhaps speech motor control processes or some combination that are associated with the disorder of stuttering. The question that arises is whether you think that the disorder of stuttering leads to these disrupted processes, subtle or gross, or do you think that perhaps these disrupted processes lead to the disorder of stuttering?

C. Mateer: I cannot think of a mechanism whereby the behavior is causing the underlying pathology. Perhaps you can give me an example.

A. Caruso: There are a number of studies, some done by people in this room, that have modified behaviors and have seen changes in neural processes underlying that same movement. On that basis there is perhaps some sort of connection between a behavior that would have an impact.

C. Mateer: Are you saying that if you modify a behavior you change the underlying neurology of it?

A. Caruso: The processes that lead to that behavior, yes.

C. Mateer: This may be unrelated, but one of the areas that I have been interested in most recently is cognitive rehabilitation and working on redevelopment of attentional processes and certain aspects of memory processing. We have been collecting data to support behavioral/cognitive changes following intervention. I feel that you can change these behaviors, increase abilities, and that differences reflect underlying change in the neural system. By providing appropriate exercise or repetition of certain behaviors I think you can redevelop and change underlying neurologic substrates.

Walter H. Moore

2   Hemispheric Processing Research
Past, Present, and Future

Introduction

Early Theories of Stuttering

Studies in the 1920s related stuttering to "shift in handedness." It was thought (q.v., Travis, 1931) that a shift from left- to right-handedness would interfere with the development of a dominant gradient of excitation in the central nervous system. L.E. Travis (1931) wrote that alterations in cortical activity and control lead to an absence of the speech dominant gradient and the subsequent outcome may be stuttering. S.T. Orton and L.E. Travis, in 1929, reported data which led to and supported this conceptualization. They stated: "We tentatively advance the suggestion that in many stutterers the motor facility as determined by training is out of harmony with the physiologic leads and this . . . fits nicely with the clinical observations of the relationship of stuttering to enforced shifts of handedness in writing in young children." They were confident that environmental factors (shift in handedness) influenced neurophysiology.

The earliest statement of a confused dominance theory was found in a 1927 article by Orton which stated: ". . . cases seem to support the theorem that stuttering . . . is often an expression of confusion in cerebral dominance. The larynx and other organs of speech, unlike the limbs, are not independent, paired organs, but are single mechanisms, though activated by paired groups of muscles on either side of the midline. The possibilities for great difficulty here through con-

39

fusion in dominance or through alternating dominance are obvious."
(Orton notes in this article that work on brain physiology with stut-
terers was started in 1925 by Travis with a Fellowship from the
National Research Council.)

Decline in Cerebral Dominance Theory

A considerable number of physiological studies were conducted during the 1920s, 1930s and 1940s to support the theory that stuttering
was related to a lack of cerebral dominance (Douglas, 1943; Freestone, 1942; Jasper, 1932; Knott and Tjossem, 1943; Lindsley, 1940;
Morley, 1935; Steer, 1937; Strother, 1935; Travis and Knott, 1936,
1937; Travis, 1934). However, during the latter part of the 1940s and
throughout the 1950s there was an obvious decline not only in "cerebral dominance" research, but also in the popularity of cerebral dominance theories to account for stuttering.

Clearly there were problems with the research that was done. The
technology was new, there was no resorting to authority for research
design, we were a new profession with little research data or laurels,
physiological research was difficult stuff at best, and the utility of
this line of research was difficult to see given the prevalent theories
of the 1950s and 1960s. All of this seems to have contributed to the
decline of hemispheric process/physiological research with a greater
emphasis placed on exploring the peripheral and social aspects of
stuttering. Williams's (1955) EMG investigation, which reported no
evidence to support the proposition that stutterers and nonstutterers
differed physiologically, also helped to reduce the interest in hemispheric processing research.

Resurgence in Hemispheric Processing

Enter R.K. Jones in 1966 with use of the Wada intracarotid amytal test
(Wada, 1949) with stutterers and a resurgence began in hemispheric
processing research with stutterers. Briefly, Jones studied four stutterers requiring operations on one cerebral hemisphere. Prior to the
operation they all demonstrated temporary "aphasic" symptoms during intracarotid amytal testing from both hemispheres. Following the
operations stuttering ceased and intracarotid amytal tests showed

speech disruption only from the side of the brain that had not been operated on. Indeed, Jones wrote: "This supports the view previously put forward, but unproved, by Travis (1931), that bilateral cortical representation is a factor in stammering."

Certainly there are concerns about the Jones study: Three of four subjects were left handed (the right-handed subject had a family history of left handedness), severity data were not provided, and the subjects had neuropathologies. With regard to the neuropathologies, with the exception of one patient with a left frontal tumour mass, all had sudden onset of subarachnoid hemorrhage. Nonetheless, these were very interesting and important data but, unfortunately, they were known to few speech-language pathologists when first published.

The study that assured the resurgence in hemispheric or cerebral dominance research was Curry and Gregory's 1969 study using dichotic procedures and published in the *Journal of Speech and Hearing Research*. At the time the study was completed dichotic procedures were relatively new (Broadbent (1954) had used them in the 1950s to look at attentional issues) and Kimura (1961a; 1961b) had recently published two papers applying the dichotic listening technique to neuropsychological issues. She suggested that the dichotic listening technique provided a noninvasive way of assessing language lateralization. We now had a new technique, with research credibility developed by psychologists, to look again at an old theory.

In essence, Curry and Gregory found that 75% of the nonstutterers obtained higher right ear scores on their dichotic verbal task, whereas 55% of the stutterers had higher left ear scores. Additionally, the between-ears difference score for the control group was more than double that for the group of stutterers on the Dichotic Word Test. The authors suggested that these ". . . differences in performance on certain dichotic listening tasks seem to reflect differences in neurophysiological organization . . . [and that they] could be interpreted as supporting a version of the theory that stutterers lack dominance. . . ." Curry and Gregory provided support for the Orton-Travis hypothesis. The data were obtained with a credible procedure that had nothing to do with speech motor activity at the periphery.

The results were not an artifact of the act of stuttering but a more direct reflection of hemispheric dominance.

Some Current Procedures and Results

Numerous studies have been done using a variety of procedures since the Jones and Curry and Gregory studies.

Dichotic Listening. The largest number of studies in the area of hemispheric processing in stutterers has been generated using this procedure. This appears to be due, in part, to the limited equipment needs and the development of computerized dichotic tapes which several laboratories and researchers have been willing to share with others. However, we need to recognize that any number of variables can affect the result obtained with dichotic procedures. These include acoustic and phonetic features of the stimuli, task, subject set, etc. (q.v., Tartter, 1988; Harshman, 1988). These variables must be carefully analyzed when comparing dichotic studies. Differences between studies may not simply be related to subject differences but to a variety of stimulus, task, and subject parameters. Indeed, dichotic word tests do not simply measure "cerebral dominance" for language (q.v., Hugdahl, 1988).

In the stuttering literature investigations that have used meaningful linguistic stimuli (that is, words) have reported a significantly larger proportion of stutterers, compared to normals, with a left ear preference (Curry and Gregory, 1969; Perrin and Eisenson, 1970; Quinn, 1972; Sommers et al., 1975; Davenport, 1979). Investigations using nonsense syllables have reported findings that are more consistent, although not completely consistent, with research involving normal populations (Cerf and Prins, 1974; Sussman and Mac-Nielage, 1975; Dorman and Porter, 1975; Brady and Berson, 1975; Pinsky and McAdam, 1980; Rosenfield and Goodglass, 1980; Liebetrau and Daly, 1981; Cimorell-Strong, Bilbert and Frick, 1983; Blood, 1985). Many of the investigations using nonsense syllables have reported a larger number of stutterers with either a left ear preference, or no ear preference score (Brady and Berson, 1975; Strong, 1978; Rosenfield and Goodglass, 1980; Liebetrau and Daly, 1981;

Cimorell-Strong et al., 1983; Blood, 1985). Perrin and Eisenson (1970) gathered data from stutterers with nonsense syllables and words. They found a left ear preference for words, but no ear preference for nonsense syllables. Results from dichotic testing using nonsense syllables have been interpreted as evidence for a "phoneme perception deficiency" (Rosenfield and Goodglass, 1980; Pinsky and McAdam, 1980) in stutterers.

Tachistoscopic Viewing. Results from visual tachistoscopic procedures with stutterers have been reported in three independent investigations (Moore, 1976; Plakosh, 1978; Hand and Haynes, 1983). These studies used meaningful linguistic stimuli, and all three found left visual half field advantages (LFA) for stutterers, implying right hemispheric activation. Nonstutterers were found to have a right visual half field advantage (RFA).

Results from tachistoscopic procedures require the same care in interpretation as do results from dichotic procedures. Findings are influenced by numerous stimulus, task, and subject variables. The studies cited all used meaningful linguistic stimuli and all found a left visual field preference in stutterers. This observation is important for a number of reasons. Most importantly, they demonstrate that differences in processing are not restricted to the auditory modality in stutterers. This observation supports a more pervasive and central mechanism associated with hemispheric processing of stutterers, reflected in the processing of both auditory and visual linguistic stimuli.

Cortical Bloodflow. This procedure is based on the observation that bloodflow through the various tissues of the body changes as a direct result of metabolic activity of the tissue (Lassen et al., 1978). Consequently, if one hemisphere or region of a hemisphere, is more or less active than another, then we expect to see differences in regional cerebral circulation.

Wood et al. (1980) used a noninvasive measurement of blood flow with two stutterers. They reported greater flow in Broca's area in the right hemisphere during stuttering. However, when the subjects were fluent greater blood flow was found in the left anterior hemisphere. This study demonstrates an important relationship between the severity of stuttering and hemispheric activation that has recently been demonstrated in two EEG studies (Boberg et al., 1983; Moore, 1986).

Evoked Potentials. There are few evoked potential studies that have been reported with stutterers. Three studies using the contingent negative variation procedure (CNV) all provide different results. Zimmerman and Knott (1974) concluded that stutterers, when processing verbal stimuli, show more variable interhemispheric relationships, and do not show a consistently larger shift in the left hemisphere than in the right. Using nonverbal stimuli and simultaneous button pushing with both thumbs in one condition, and the utterance of the same fluently spoken word in another condition, Pinsky and McAdam (1980) concluded that their results, using the CNV method, provided insufficient evidence to support hemispheric asymmetry differences between stutterers and nonstutterers. Prescott and Andrews (1984) found greater right CNV's in both stutterers and nonstutterers and suggested that more attention needed to be paid to the nature of the response in CNV research.

Using meaningful words embedded in phrases to evoke average evoked responses Ponsford, Brown, Marsh and Travis (1975) found greater AER's over the right hemisphere in normals and over the left in stutterers.

That there are so few evoked potential studies with stutterers may be a reflection that both the equipment and knowledge base needed to conduct this type of electrophysiological research are typically not available to speech-language pathologists in training programs and clinics.

Hemispheric Alpha Asymmetries. Numerous studies (Galin and Ornstein, 1972; Haynes and Moore, 1981; McKee, Humphrey and McAdam, 1973; Moore and Haynes, 1980; Morgan, MacDonald and MacDonald, 1971; Robbins and McAdam, 1974) have shown increased suppression of alphabrain wave (8–13 Hz) amplitude over the hemisphere which is primarily involved in processing specific kinds of information under specific task conditions. Differential suppression of alpha activity has been the basis for claims of functional asymmetry. One of the advantages of the hemispheric alpha procedure is that it has excellent temporal resolution. That is, the researcher is able to monitor brain activity over time and observe differences in alpha activity. The procedure is not without its problems. However, if your research questions deal with the dynamic activation of the brain while processing and performing cognitive tasks, then recording spontaneous EEG can be a very helpful procedure. As with evoked potential research, few speech-language pathologists have been involved with research using spontaneous EEG. Again, this appears in part to reflect the knowledge base and equipment needs required.

Moore and his associates (Moore, 1986; Moore, 1984; Moore, Craven and Faber, 1982; Moore and Haynes, 1980; Moore and Lang, 1977; Ray and Moore, 1989; Wells and Moore, 1989), using the EEG hemispheric alpha asymmetry procedure, have consistently reported greater alpha suppression in the right posterior temporal-parietal area in male stutterers using meaningful linguistic stimuli (high and low imagery words, and connected discourse) under conditions of recall and recognition. Boberg, Yeudall, Schopflocher and Bo-Lassen (1983) have found greater alpha suppression in the right posterior frontal brain areas of stutterers prior to clinical management. Following clinical management which increased fluency these investigators reported a shift in hemispheric alpha suppression to the left posterior frontal area. This observation suggests that gains in fluency that are obtained with clinical management produce a change in the processing strategies employed by the stutterer to establish and maintain fluent speech, as reflected in a shift from right to left hemispheric alpha suppression. In support of this finding, Moore (1984) reported right hemispheric alpha suppression during baseline with a gradual and consistent suppression of left hemispheric alpha as stuttering decreased using biofeedback (EMG) in a single subject experimental design.

Moore (1986) observed a negative relationship between measures of stuttering and hemispheric alpha ratios obtained during recall tasks. These data indicate that as the frequency of stuttering increases, right hemispheric alpha decreases during active tasks requiring verbal recall but not recognition. More severe stutterers tend to have greater right hemisphere activation during recall tasks. These data suggest that hemispheric activation in stutterers is not a dichotomous variable but rather a continuous one, with greater stuttering related to greater degrees of right hemispheric activation during recall tasks.

Two recent investigations conducted in our laboratory (Ray and Moore, 1989; Wells and Moore, 1989) have not found differences between stutterers and nonstutterers during resting conditions with the absence of linguistic stimuli. Differences in hemispheric activation between these two groups were found only during active linguistic tasks. These data imply that differences observed between stutterers and nonstutterers are not related to differences in brain morphology but rather to cognitive modes of information processing.

Future Concerns and Conclusions

There is much to be accomplished in the area of hemispheric processing with changes in technology with a variety of speech and language disorders including stuttering. Our EEG procedures will be changing in the weeks ahead to include brain electrical activity mapping (Duffy, 1981). With this system we will be able to gather 20 channels of spontaneous EEG as well as 20 channels of visual and/or auditory evoked potentials. One of the important features of the cortical topography procedure is that it allows you to analyze large amounts of electrophysiological data and display the data in cortical maps for specific segments of the signal epoch. I am particularly interested in evoked potential data with stutterers as related to attentional and cognitive strategies. This new technology will allow us to look at hemispheric processing and function in greater detail and increase both our spatial and temporal resolution. Thus, our research questions and investigations can begin to take a different look at hemispheric processing in stutterers.

There are numerous areas of concern in hemispheric processing research with stutterers. One of the greatest concerns for me is the interpretation of hemispheric processing data. We need to look closely at our models of hemispheric processing derived from the data we gather. In the fixed trait model (Harshman, 1988) patterns of cerebral functional specialization are presumed to be relatively invariant characteristics of the human species. With this kind of a model an experimental nonreplication would clearly indicate that one or the other researcher is in error. Many laterality researchers and consumers of laterality research seem to operate under this model of brain organization. Clearly, this model does not account for the empirical data that have shown variation associated with stimulus effects, tasks effects, and subject effects (including handedness and sex). According to Harshman: "If there are many different patterns of cognitive abilities, then perhaps such natural variation in brain organization, in interaction with environmental factors, underlies much of the natural variation in cognitive ability patterns that we see in the human population. . . . This alternative to the 'fixed species trait' model might be called the 'individual differences'." An individual differences model more elegantly accounts for the variations found in the neuropsychological literature. Unfortunately, many practitioners and academicians in speech-language pathology have not been exposed to the voluminous data that supports an individual differences model. All too often we have been exposed to an antiquated cerebral dominance model of brain function (left/language, right/nonlanguage) that was developed in the mid 1800s. The idea of a rigid dichotomy of function or of one half of the brain being "dominant" for something is an outmoded concept and is not supported by empirical data. The concept of processing does not imply "dominance" of one hemisphere over another, but simply suggests a mode of information processing which one or the other hemispheres is more suited, morphologically and cognitively, to engage in than the other. If decisions about hemispheric processing research are to be made relative to its implications for theory and therapy they must be made with a complete and unbiased knowledge of all the relevant empirical data and current theory. The benefactors of data based decisions are the individuals that suffer from fluency disorders.

Stuttered verbal behavior is the outcome of a neurophysiological process. What we observe at the behavioral periphery is not the process itself but rather the outcome of the process. Medical science (and speech-language pathology) has a long history of being led up dead ends when we study only peripheral symptoms. Symptoms accompany disease processes but they are not the disease itself. Disorders such as epilepsy and diabetes could never have been managed if we dealt only with the behavioral manifestations of the disease processes. If we are to understand peripheral behaviors associated with stuttering we must aggressively investigate the neurophysiological process of which they are an outcome. As with other disease/disorder processes, this does not imply that we stop managing behavior. It implies that what we manage may change drastically once we understand the process of which the symptom is an outcome. (Behavioral management of polyuria will do little to manage diabetes. Dietary behavioral management does help in the management of diabetes. Yet, this was not known until the process of diabetes was understood.) The focus of behavioral management can change when we understand the process causing the symptom. We are close to understanding the process of which stuttered verbal behavior is the outcome. Before the implications of neurophysiological research in stuttering become a practical reality we will have to shed many unuseful theories and preconceived notions about stuttering and address ourselves to empirical issues in an informed manner.

References

Blood, G. (1985). Laterality differences in child stutterers: Heterogeneity, severity levels, and statistical treatment. *Journal of Speech and Hearing Disorders* 50: 66–72.

Boberg, E., Yeudall, L., Schopflocher, D., and Bo-Lassen, P. (1983). The effect of an intensive behavioral program on the distribution of EEG alpha power in stutterers during the processing of verbal and visuospatial information. *Journal of Fluency Disorders* 8: 245–63.

Broadbent, D.E. (1954). The role of auditory localization in attention and memory span. *Journal of Experimental Psychology* 47: 191–96.

Brady, J.P. and Berson, J. (1975). Stuttering, dichotic listening and cerebral dominance. *Archives of General Psychiatry* 32: 1449–59.

Cerf, A. and Prins, D. (1974). Stutterers' ear preference for dichotic syllables. Paper presented to the Annual Convention of the American Speech and Hearing Association, Las Vegas.

Cimorell-Strong, J.M., Gilbert, H.R. and Frick, J.V. (1983). Dichotic speech perception: A comparison between stuttering and nonstuttering children. *Journal of Fluency Disorders* 8: 77–91.

Curry, F. and Gregory, H. (1969). The performance of stutterers on dichotic listening tasks thought to reflect cerebral dominance. *Journal of Speech and Hearing Research* 12: 73–82.

Davenport, R.W. (1979). Dichotic listening in four severity levels of stuttering. *ASHA* 21: 769 (abstract).

Dorman, M.F. and Porter, R.J., Jr. (1975). Hemispheric lateralization for speech perception in stutterers. *Cortex* 11: 181–85.

Douglass, L.C. (1943). A study of bilaterally recorded electroencephalograms of adult stutterers. *Journal of Experimental Psychology* 32: 247–65.

Duffy, F.H. (1981). Brain electrical activity mapping (BEAM): Computerized access to complex brain function. *International Journal of Neuroscience* 13: 55–65.

Freestone, N.W. (1942). An electroencephalographic study on the moment of stuttering. *Speech Monographs* 9: 28–60.

Galin, D. and Ornstein, R. (1972). Lateral specialization of cognitive modes: An EEG study. *Psychophysiology* 9: 412–18.

Hand, C.R. and Hanes, W.O. (1983). Linguistic processing and reaction time differences in stutterers and nonstutterers. *Journal of Speech and Hearing Research* 26: 181–85.

Harshman, R.A. (1988). Dichotic listening assessment of group and individual differences: Methodological and practical issues. In Hugdahl, K., ed., *Handbook of Dichotic Listening*. New York: John Wiley and Sons.

Haynes, W.O. and Moore, W.H., Jr. (1981a). Sentence imagery and recall: An electroencephalographic evaluation of hemispheric processing in males and females. *Cortex* 17: 49–62.

———. (1981b). Recognition and recall: An electroencephalographic investigation of hemispheric alpha asymmetries for males and females on perceptual and retrieval tasks. *Perceptual and Motor Skills* 53: 283–90.

Hugdahl, K., ed., (1988). *Handbook of dichotic listening: Theory, methods and research*. New York: John Wiley and Sons.

Jasper, H.H. (1932). A laboratory study of diagnostic indices of bilateral neuromuscular organization in stutterers and normal speakers. *Psychology Monographs* 43: 72–174.

Jones, R.K. (1966). Observations on stammering after localized cerebral injury. *Journal of Neurology, Neurosurgery and Psychiatry* 29: 192–95.

Kimura, D. (1961a). Some effects of temporal-lobe damage on auditory perception. *Canadian Journal of Psychology* 15: 156–65.

———. (1961b). Cerebral dominance and the perception of verbal stimuli. *Canadian Journal of Psychology* 15: 166–75.

Knott, J.R. and Tjossem, T.D. (1943). Bilateral electroencephalograms from normal speakers and stutterers. *Journal of Experimental Psychology* 32: 357–62.

Lassen, N.A., Ingvar, D.H. and Skinhoj, E. (1978). Brain function and blood flow. *Scientific American* 239: 62–71.

Liebetrau, R.M. and Daly, D.A. (1981). Auditory processing and perceptual abilities of "organic" and "functional" stutterers. *Journal of Fluency Disorders* 6: 219–31.

Lindsley, D.B. (1940). Bilateral differences in brain potentials from the two cerebral hemispheres in relation to laterality and stuttering. *Journal of Experimental Psychology* 26: 211–25.

McKee, G., Humphrey, B. and McAdam, D. (1973). Scaled lateralizations of alpha activity during linguistic and musical tasks. *Psychophysiology* 10: 441–43.

Moore, W.H., Jr. (1976). Bilateral tachistoscopic word perception of stutterers and normal subjects. *Brain and Language* 3: 434–42.

———. (1984). Hemispheric alpha asymmetries during an electromyographic biofeedback procedure for stuttering: A single-subject experimental design. *Journal of Fluency Disorders* 17: 143–62.

———. (1986). Hemispheric alpha asymmetries of stutterers and nonstutterers for the recall and recognition of words and connected reading passages: Some relationships to severity of stuttering. *Journal of Fluency Disorders* 11: 71–89.

Moore, W.H., Jr. and Boberg, E. (1987). Hemispheric processing and stuttering. In Rustin , L., Purser, H. and Rowley, D., eds., *Progress in the Treatment of Fluency Disorders*. London: Taylor and Francis.

Moore, W.H., Jr., Craven, D.C. and Faber, M. (1982). Hemispheric alpha asymmetries of words with positive, negative, and neutral arousal values preceding tasks of recall and recognition: Electrophysiological and behavioral results from stuttering males and nonstuttering males and females. *Brain and Language* 17: 211–24.

Moore, W.H., Jr. and Haynes, W.O. (1980a). Alpha hemispheric asymmetry and stuttering: Some support for a segmentation dysfunction hypothesis. *Journal of Speech and Hearing Research* 23: 229–47.

————. (1980b). A study of alpha hemispheric asymmetries and their relationship to verbal and nonverbal abilities in males and females. *Brain and Language* 9: 338–49.

Moore, W.H., Jr. and Lang, M.K. (1977). Alpha asymmetry over the right and left hemispheres of stutterers and control subjects preceding massed oral readings: A preliminary investigation. *Perceptual and Motor Skills* 44: 223–30.

Moore, W.H., Jr. and Lorendo, L. (1980). Alpha hemispheric asymmetries of stuttering and nonstuttering subjects for words of high and low imagery. *Journal of Fluency Disorders* 5: 11–26.

Morgan, S.H., McDonald, P.J. and MacDonald, H. (1971). Differences in bilateral alpha activity as a function of experimental tasks with a note on lateral eye movements and hypnotizability. *Neuropsychologia* 9: 459–69.

Morley, A.J. (1935). An analysis of the associative and predisposing factors in the symptomatology of stuttering. Ph.D. Dissertation, State University of Iowa.

Orton, S.T. (1927). Studies in stuttering. *Archives of Neurology and Psychiatry* 18: 671–72.

Orton, S.T. and Travis, L.E. (1929). Studies in stuttering: IV. Studies of action currents in stutterers. *Archives of Neurology and Psychiatry* 21: 61–68.

Perrin, K.L. and Eisenson, J. (1970). An examination of ear preference for speech and nonspeech stimuli in a stuttering population. Paper presented at the Annual Convention of the American Speech and Language Association, New York.

Pinsky, S.D. and McAdam, D.W. (1980). Electroencephalographic and dichotic indices of cerebral laterality in stutterers. *Brain and Language* 11: 374–97.

Plakosh, P. (1978). The functional asymmetry of the brain: Hemispheric specialization in stutterers for processing of visually presented linguistic and spatial stimuli. Unpublished doctoral dissertation, the Palo Alto School of Professional Psychology.

Ponsford, R., Brown, W., Marsh, J. and Travis, L. (1975). Evoked potential correlates of cerebral dominance for speech perception in stutterers and nonstutterers. *Electroencephalography and Clinical Neurophysiology* 39: 434 (abstract).

Prescott, J. and Andrews, G. (1984). Early and late components of the contingent negative variation prior to manual and speech responses in stutterers and nonstutterers. *International Journal of Psychophysiology* 2: 121–30.

Quinn, P.T. (1972). Stuttering, cerebral dominance and the dichotic word test. *Medical Journal of Australia* 2: 639–43.

Ray, D. and Moore, W.H., Jr. (1990). Effect of perception, formulation and production during a quasi-conversational task: An EEG alpha asymmetry investigation of male stutterers and male and female nonstutterers. *Journal of Neurolinguistics* 3: 1–21.

Robbins, K.I. and McAdam, D.W. (1974). Interhemispheric alpha asymmetry and imagery mode. *Brain and Language* 1: 189–93.

Rosenfield, D.B. and Goodglass, H. (1980). Dichotic testing of cerebral dominance in stutterers. *Brain and Language* 11: 170–80.

Sommers, R.K., Brady, W. and Moore, W.H., Jr. (1975). *Perceptual and Motor Skills* 41: 931–38.

Spellacy, F. and Blumstein, S. (1970). The influence of language set on ear preference in phoneme recognition. *Cortex* 6: 430–39.

Steer, M. (1937). Symptomatologies of young stutterers. *Journal of Speech Disorders* 2: 3–13.

Strong, J.C. (1978). Dichotic speech perception: a comparison between stutterers and nonstutterers. *ASHA* 20: 728 (abstract).

Strother, C.A. (1935). A study of the extent of dysynergia occurring during the stuttering spasm. Ph.D. Dissertation, State University of Iowa.

Sussman, H.M. and MacNeilage, P.F. (1975). Hemispherid specialization for speech production and perception in stutterers. *Neuropsychologia* 9: 19–26.

Tartter, V. (1988). Acoustic and phonetic feature effects in dichotic listening scores. In Hugdahl, K., ed., *Handbook of dichotic listening: Theory, methods and research*. New York: John Wiley and Sons.

Travis, L.E. (1934). Dissociation of the homologous muscle function in stuttering. *Archives of Neurology and Psychiatry* 31: 127–33.

———. (1931). *Speech Pathology*. New York: Appleton-Century-Crofts.

Travis, L.E. and Knott, J.R. (1936). Brain potentials from normal speakers and stutterers. *Journal of Psychology* 2: 137–50.

———. (1937). Bilaterally recorded brain potentials from normal speakers and stutterers. *Journal of Speech Disorders* 2: 239–41.

Wada, J.A. (1949). A new method for the determination of the side of cerebral speech dominance. *Medical Biology* 14: 221–22.

Wells, B. and Moore, W.H., Jr. (1990). EEG alpha asymmetries in stutterers and nonstutterers: Effects of linguistic variables on hemispheric processing and fluency. *Neuropsychologia* 28: 1295–1305.

Williams, D.E. (1955). Masseter muscle action potentials in stuttered and nonstuttered speech. *Journal of Speech and Hearing Disorders* 20: 242–61.

Wood, F., Stump, D., McKeehan, A., Sheldon, S. and Proctor, J. (1980). Patterns of regional cerebral blood flow during attempted reading aloud by stutterers both on and off haloperiodol medication: Evidence for inadequate left frontal activation during stuttering. *Brain and Language* 9: 141–44.

Zimmerman, G.N. and Knott, J.R. (1974). Slow potentials of the brain in relation to speech processing in normal speakers and stutterers. *Electroencephalography and Clinical Neurophysiology* 37: 599–607.

Discussion

A. Rochet: The first question that our group would like to pose has to do with the use of alpha wave suppression and regional blood flow techniques. How do you determine that the observed differences that you see between stutterers and nonstutterers on these two procedures are a function of language processing differences and not some sort of right hemisphere activity difference associated with emotional or affective instability?

W. Moore: Let me tell you that some of the data that my colleague, Betsy G. Wells, who has collaborated with me in this area of research for several years, presented indicated that during a "rest position," when subjects are told to concentrate on breathing, there were no differences in left and right hemisphere alpha suppression between normals and stutterers. Nobody had any suppression that was significant over the left or right hemisphere. They were the same. Now that is not to say that when you put somebody in a room, and say, "now rest and don't think about anything," that they all do that. That is a problem and you need to recognize that.

Typically we tell subjects to go into the room, concentrate on breathing and get them to relax. Then we take the recordings. When we did that in two recent investigations we found no differences between normals and stutterers in terms of hemispheric activation. Differences that were found, in terms of hemisphere activation, appeared only during the presentation of the linguistic stimuli. At that point we found activation differences between the groups and we inferred differences in terms of the way they were processing information. Obviously we are physiologizing here, no question about it. We have published research, I showed you some of those data, where we have asked subjects what they were doing during the tasks they were asked to do. They reported a variety of different procedures. We forced some of the subjects into a dichotomy, in terms of visualizing and auditorizing information. We found differences in those subjects which we then inferred to indicate that the mode of processing was importantly related to the differences we found in hemispheric asymmetry. I do not think that it is anything that is hard wired in terms of stutterers or normals for that matter. I think it is the way they approach problem solving. It sounds kind of general but I do not know how to conceptualize it beyond that. How does one solve the problem? What kind of strategies do they use? There is a lot more to be done in that area.

A. Rochet: Obviously, there are some task differences that affect the hemispheric activation patterns across conditions, whether subjects are listening to speech, thinking about speaking, or actually speaking, and within the speaking conditions whether they are speaking fluently or nonfluently. Could you comment on some of the methodological issues associated with such experimental ambiguities? For example, what are the temporal limits of your sampling windows, and might they be contaminated by dysfluent moments within a fluent period?

W. Moore: There are a lot of problems with the research. Any time you stick an electrode on somebody and begin to deal with amplifiers you are going to have problems with all kinds of artifacts. Let me talk about task differences for a minute and then get down to the production thing. The fact of the matter is that I have really done very few investigations that deal with production. The reason is that when you begin to get a subject involved with production tasks you are going to get EMGs spilling over into the EEG. You are concerned about that and you do not want any artifact. You can set your filters, transistorized filters, but there are still some concerns about what may be going on there. For that reason, the vast majority of research that I have done has dealt with perceptual kinds of tasks. Betsy reported on an investigation where we looked at production tasks. It is conceivable that some of those data are contaminated by what the stutterer was actually doing during those tasks. There is no question about that. I am still impressed with the fact that there are differences in the alpha frequency for normals and stutterers for those tasks. It is not just a matter of EMG spilling over into the EEG.

Now if the question is, could there be more muscle activity in the stutterers because they are stuttering, that is another question. The answer is yes, it could be. It definitely could be. Could that account for the differences? It might, but I am not aware of any empirical data that says that it does. My data seemed to support the idea that the same kinds of things are being found with the perceptual task. It is interesting to note that some of the stuff we showed indicated that you see less of it during production tasks than you do during perceptual tasks. You see less right hemispheric activation on the ratio data. We saw that pretty clearly: the line moved towards the center. On the production data that Betsy showed we only got the production effect with stutterers when we went to the simple effects analysis to get rid of some of the other variance from the normals. Then we began to get the production effect. But on the main analysis of all the variables we did not get a production effect for stutterers. When we forced it by dropping a variable and looking at it through a simple effects model then it began to arise. I have often been concerned about why we do not find anterior differences with stutterers during some of our tasks. Now that does not totally answer your question but it is a methodological issue. I am ready to look at any data that would suggest better ways to control that. I am aware of the problems of this research.

A. Rochet: Our group was interested in the individual variation that you might have found within the stuttering group itself. We would also appreciate some comment about gender distribution within the stuttering group, if both sexes were represented.

W. Moore: I do not do research with stutterers by just grouping them all together as males and females. I have not done that in years for the obvious reason that there is a sex ratio difference and there must be something going on there. We have not had enough female stutterers to fill up a group so I have done these unbalanced designs with nonstuttering males, nonstuttering females and stuttering males. We have used nonstuttering females because the literature in sex research and hemispheric processing research does show differences with female and male nonstutterers. We wanted to get some comparisons between stutterers and females and males to see if we could discern some differences between those two normal groups that we could not see in the stuttering males. There is no distribution there. We have not done much research with females. Not because I do not want to do it, not because I do not think it is a good thing to do. I think it is an important thing to do but we have not had the subjects to fit into those categories for one reason or another.

A. Rochet: Then within the male stuttering group what was the individual variation?

W. Moore: One of the variables that has to be accounted for here is the severity of stuttering. What are they doing during the time this stuff is going on, in terms of their fluency? I have found that with any kind of a "pathological group," be it an aphasic or a stutterer, that there is less variability in the pathological group than there is in the normal group. I wondered about that for awhile. What is going on here? Why do we find less variability in this group? It seems to me that a normal individual, who does not stutter or have aphasia or a language disorder, has many more information processing strategies available to him or her. They can bounce back and forth between left and right strategies all the time. We do it all the time. There is no question about it. Our research with normals has clearly indicated that. We find a lot of variability in normal groups. When it comes to stutterers, one of the things we have to deal with is that the relationship between hemispheric processing and stuttering becomes stronger with a greater severity in stuttering. We begin to talk about "subgroups," and a lot of folks seem to say we found a subgroup that seems to be doing this and a sub-group that seems to be doing that, but nobody seems to talk about the level of dysfluency. If it is a continuum that has some-thing to do with the way they access the brain, then it is not a matter of a subgroup. It is just more of something within the group. I am convinced that if we do not look at how much stut-tering is going on, which means how they process information differently, then we are going to continue to get variance. There is variance but that variance is not necessarily greater than the variance one would expect to find within the normal group. In fact, many times it is less. That variance can be controlled, by looking at severity, either by grouping subjects differently or by statistical control.

M. Neilson: The number one question that I want to ask has to do with something that you mentioned and emphasized a couple of times through your talk; that it is necessary in any of this sort of testing to pay attention to task demands. Am I right? Now we were discussing in our group a study which came out of Edwards Air Force base of the U.S. Military. It measured the differential activation of the hemispheres of pilots in a real life situation, not a simulated situation. There was a real plane and a computer in the plane with complete monitoring. When these guys went up, their hemispheric activation, by means of alpha and theta power suppression, was looked at in a normal task performance situation when the plane was flying and the pilot was completely in control of it. It was also looked at when some people pulled some tricks on that pilot that made the plane uncontrollable. They had a look at his hemispheric activation patterns when he was trying to get out of a potentially very uncontrollable situation. They saw the differential patterns of the hemispheric activation during the controlled situation. During the situation of very high task demand it fell to virtually equal pattern of hemispheric activation. We discussed this and wondered about the implications for the things that you are presenting on stuttering.*

W. Moore: I have not the vaguest idea what those implications are. The empirical data that we have gathered with stutterers and normals have shown that on recognition and recall tasks there are differences in hemispheric activation, certainly with normals. We have consistently found that with recall tasks there is greater left hemispheric activation, not surprisingly, than in

---

* The study I was referring to is that of Sterman et al., (1988) who report data from both in-flight and simulator performance. Playing "tricks" on pilots is only appropriate in simulator studies and, in discussing the in-flight data, I misquoted the method but not the result. I should have said that hemispheric activation was examined during competent performance and also during times when the pilot was in circumstances that made it difficult to control the aircraft, for instance, during a verified period of spatial disorientation. During competent performance the data from these real tasks, as well as from the flight simulator studies, showed significant discrepancies between the hemispheres in activation in the alpha range. In contrast, during poor or failed performance, this differential activation was attenuated or abolished.

Sterman, M.B., Schummer, G.J., Dushenko, T.W. & Smith, J.C. (1988). Electroencephalographic correlates of pilot performance: Simulation and in-flight studies. In *Conference Proceedings No. 432, North Atlantic Treaty Organization, Advisory Group for Aerospace Research and Development (AGARD)*, Neuilly sur Seine, France, pp. 31–1 to 31–16.

recognition tasks where there is stimulus support. So on those two cognitive tasks, different things seem to be going on in the person's brain relative to the stimulus support that is provided, relative to the kinds of information they have to do to dredge up.

I have never done anything with anybody on an airplane flying at Mach 1, 2, or 3 and I do not know how to address your question except to get involved with some fantasy about what may have been going on there. The important thing to recognize is that if we conceptualize the brain as processing in a lateral mode only we are making a mistake. I suspect that when one is placed in a crisis situation, let us assume those tricks represented that to the pilot, and if that plane is going to go down, you have to resort to many different strategies in order to overcome the risks. If one does not work then you go to another. I think that a normal brain is far better at doing that than one that is using only a limited number of strategies, like an aphasic or a stutterer who might be locked into a stuttering mode at the time. I think it may have any number of implications but I really do not know. It may well be that the individual is accessing many different kinds of problem solving strategies at the time of the trick and that may be very, very important. That seems to me to say that it is left brain, right brain, left brain, right brain. It is not a matter of lateralization. We have got to begin to look at cognitive variables. Who cares about physiological data if you do not have a behavioral correlate? Certainly not me. It does not mean anything. We have been trapped by physiologizing before. What was that person doing? What did the individual have to do? When did the brain wave pattern appear to be the same? When was it different? When was it left, when right, when bilateral? Those are the kinds of questions that I would be concerned about. Not so much that they found no difference during the trick segment of the experiment but what was the subject doing.

M. Neilson: Would it be fair to say that during that crisis situation the person presumably is short on resources to cope with the situation adequately and that in a situation where you are short on resources you pull them in from everywhere? Perhaps stutterers are short on resources for certain speech-language based tasks and in fact are pulling them from anywhere that they can. Therefore, we see a more equal pattern of activation.

W. Moore: I would agree with that interpretation, a whole lot. That is conceivable. I do not know if it is true, but it is conceivable.

M. Neilson: We would like you to elaborate on how stutterers should approach their cognitive tasks differently from how they customarily do. What cognitive task should we be focusing on, how might you bring that about and what are the eventual implications for treatment?

W. Moore: There are a number of variables that I think you have to look at in stuttering before answering that question directly. First of all it is no coincidence that the locus of stuttering seems to be based on what the right hemisphere seems to be able to process linguistically and what it can not. There seems to be no mistake that stutterers have a worse time of it when they are using passive sentences than when they are using active sentences. Research seems to indicate that the right hemisphere is not good at dealing with syntactic structuredness such as in passive sentences. It seems to be no mistake that stutterers do better at processing high visual imagery information than low visual imagery information. There seems to be no mistake that stutterers do better with transition times that are longer than shorter and that the left hemisphere is really good at processing short transitional information, particularly the duration of time between first and second format transitions. When you begin to look at plosives, for instance, you find that there are real short transition times. When a stutterer says "I have a lot of problems with plosives," it does not surprise me.

When you begin to look at all these linguistic variables you begin to wonder why stuttering occurs with greater probability at phrase boundaries and not within phrase boundaries. What does that have to do with hemispheric processing? Well, it has a lot to do with it. How come they do better with voicing than unvoicing? Voicing is processed differently in the brain than is place of articulation. Why are there differences in that regard? It looks to me to be yet another reflection of how the stutterer is processing information. When they are stuttering there is a difference in processing. What do we do then? It is easy to say that you have to make them more segmental, more left hemispheric and you have to get them involved with what transitions are. You have to get them involved with what phrase structure rules are. I suspect that if you took a few paragraphs without any punctuation, gave them to some stutterers and said, "show me the phrases here," you might find some interesting things, particularly when they are dysfluent. They might have difficulties dealing with that phraseology. It may then be that the treatment is to get the stutterer to be more segmental. I do not know what is pushing this thing.

Now the interesting thing is that we do have a couple of ways of approaching this issue therapeutically. We can play the right hemisphere. We can do what the right hemisphere does best. It deals with slow transitions (spoken in a prolonged manner) and that plays right into what the right hemisphere says, "I can deal with that," and stutterers do deal with that. They do not stay fluent that way very long. The hard part is getting them to talk like nonstutterers. Getting them to use proper transitions. Those therapy procedures that have done that have been real successful and the stutterers end up loving their clinicians. They do not burn out, things are working well and things are happening. We do not have enough data on what's going on physiologically in those kinds of therapeutic procedures.

I am convinced that masking, DAF and syllable timed speech, etc., only intensify the problem the stutterer has, which is the utilization of right hemispheric processing strategies. If you stretch out the transitions for the stutterers you are not doing them any favors. You are getting this strange speech out of them. They do not like it, you do not like it and everybody says "you are weird." Our problem as clinicians is in making the transition shorter.

One particular success that I had, working with nothing but phraseology and transition time, was a severe stutterer who had been told that it was a cross he would have to bear all his life. Maybe that is true but when we dealt with phraseology and transitions, that person got fluent and managed to stay fluent. We did not deal so much with stuttering per se but we went through long programs describing what a phrase is and is not and what phrases do and do not do. We explained that we use phrases for coherent communication of information, both as speakers and as listeners, which seems to be true. The smallest unit of language is a phrase, not the syllable. He was able to intellectualize what was going on and that seemed to work. I am convinced that there is clinical utility in this. I am also convinced that some of the programs that have worked very well with stutterers have done all of the right things in terms of dealing with those rapid transitions.

I think we have to look at the left hemisphere. That left hemisphere is important. It involves not only production of rapid transitions but also the perception of those rapid transitions. If the research is correct that has been done on the planum temporale we should watch how it is importantly involved in the perception of rapid transitions. If we add that to what seems to be going on with Broca's area and its importance for rapid transitions, it comes together very nicely. If you then want to say that the pulvinar connects the anterior and posterior language areas of the brain, all of a sudden we have one huge mechanism. Not two or three separate mechanisms, but one mechanism that allows us to deal with language out of the common deep structure. That is not too new. It comes from Canadians Penfield and Roberts at McGill University. There are a lot of things that this points to; those therapeutic procedures that deal with segmentation, recognition and realization of what phrase markers are, etc.

M. Neilson: We next started discussing applications of this research to measurement with children. We understand there are rumors that you will be doing some work with children? People were keen for you to give some brief comments on that. Someone specifically asked whether you envisage that by identifying a normalized pattern of hemispheric activation in children you might be able to pick out those who are at special risk for ongoing chronic language disorder or stuttering. Somebody even went so far as to ask whether you reckon that, way down the line, one might be able to incorporate such testing into a nice little black box that one could take and use in school districts?

W. Moore: Definitely, and I am going to patent it. We did some early research on children with dichotic listening. Gordon Blood also did some dichotic studies with children. The interesting thing that came from both of those dichotic investigations was that the children showed the right hemispheric effect more than the adults and the adolescents. We did our dichotic investigation with children in about 1972, and Gordon published his investigation in 1984 or 1985. There was a long time between investigations so there does seem to be something there with children. At the Northwestern conference I resolved to go back and do some research with children but that resolve has not been realized yet.

We have begun to do some research with Bruce Ryan and the children in his project. I stopped gathering the data for this reason. My data have convinced me that you are not going to get an effect unless there is stuttering. With the children that Dr. Ryan was using I saw very little dysfluency. We are not going to get an effect unless there is some stuttering. Those were not stuttering children. We were getting no place fast with those data.

That brings up one of the problems in the data which is not my problem or Bruce's problem. It is that those children present yet another problem that we have to deal with. Stuttering seems to be a little more cyclical in those children and the research has to be designed accordingly. The research I got involved with was just slapping some electrodes on a child. It was not a very good research design. Should we look at children when they are fluent and then when they are dysfluent? That makes sense to me. Do we look at them at separate times? Yes. If it is reported in the environment that there is a period of high dysfluency in the child maybe we need to run that child. If there is a time when there is low dysfluency reported in the child then we need to run that child again. With the children that I have seen, we ran eight or ten children, I did not hear one stutter. My data convince me that if you are not stuttering you look like a nonstutterer, in terms of hemispheric processing, but when you are stuttering you look like a stutterer.

M. Neilson: Dr. Moore, we have two more questions. One concerns the experimental controls in the testing that you have done. The other question concerns your interpretations of differing activations that you have seen. But I think if we hold those questions and give the third discussant a turn, perhaps there will be time to get back to them.

K. Burk: I would like to begin by thanking you for an excellent presentation. Our group was delighted, although inundated with data. Do you feel that we will in some way be able to identify subgroups of stutterers? Will we need to look at variables other than those that we clearly define as subgroups of speakers?

W. Moore: Without talking about anybody who has "neurological stuttering" I think there is a continuum. We are seeing that when the severity of stuttering is greater there is more right hemispheric activation in those stutterers. We have to get into what the microvariable, severity of stuttering, means: whatever increases it; whatever keeps it going. We need to look at those variables in order to begin to identify what is happening in terms of processing. That is a big job. This is not a cop-out but all of you who have done stuttering research and clinical work know that it takes a huge amount of time to analyze what is going on. Then we also are concerned about our reliability, etc.

I was real happy that the NIH had a conference on stuttering and is funding more research. Hopefully, that means that the political tide and our improved research designs will get us more funding from the federal government so that we can accomplish some of these things. There just has not been much funding from the federal government for stuttering research for the past number of years. We as a profession have got to do something about that. I am convinced that the NIH is now in a posture to encourage and help get that research done.

K. Burk: Could you share with us some of the characteristics of the stutterers that you have used as subjects. We had a number of questions in terms of severity level, duration and number of treatment methods. One question in particular was whether the stutterers were attempting to control speech during any of the data collection.

W. Moore: All good questions. We have mentioned in several articles that a variety of therapeutic techniques had been used on these stutterers in the past. We thought that would be a variable that could influence our data. We mentioned that some had been worked up on the Monterey program and some had been worked up on DAF. We did not quite know what that variable was doing with our subjects. When it came to severity of stuttering, we had a variety of different levels of severity. I suspect that our stutterers, like most populations of stutterers, tend towards the moderate to the mild-moderate level in terms of severity with some more severe ones sprinkled in. In order to deal with that we used correlational procedures to look at alpha symmetry and our measures of dysfluency. That is the only way we have looked at it. We have not grouped subjects in terms of severity level. I think it would be important to group subjects, by levels of severity, if you could come up with the right matrix. I do not know if all of my subjects were attempting to control stuttering or not. I suspect some of them were, no question about that. I suspect that the procedure that was used in terms of getting them fluent may have had some effect upon what we were observing in terms of hemispheric processing data. Lots of questions to be answered.

M. Neilson: We did have some discussion on the interpretations of the Alberta study on measurement of alpha suppression and your own studies. As we discussed it we concluded that both studies had shown a shift in activation from right to left. Does that mean that the processing is shifting or does it mean that the left hemisphere was doing O.K. in the stutterer but the right hemisphere was previously interfering with it? I am talking specifically about the Alberta study where the stutterers were tested before and after treatment and a shift was seen. We wondered if you might give us your interpretation of that result because I believe that the Alberta interpretation was that the right hemisphere had been interfering with the processing of the left hemisphere which now is freed to do its own processing.

W. Moore: I have no difficulties with that interpretation whatsoever. It may well be interference. If the right hemisphere is more active than the left hemisphere in programming a particular motor task that would certainly interfere with the left hemisphere's ability. I think that the importance of those data is that, like the blood flow investigation, they showed that there were different things going on during stuttering compared to more fluent speech. We replicated that, in part, with our feedback investigation. I tend not to use the term interference although I do not have a problem with the term. I keep thinking in terms of greater utilization of the less efficient right hemispheric processing strategies during stuttering and greater utilization of more efficient left hemispheric motor processing strategies during fluency. You can call that interference if you like and it may well be. I do not know what the mechanism of interference is. Is it a gating mechanism in terms of the thalmus? Is one pulvinar not being properly innervated by the reticular activating system and consequently shunting stuff to the right instead of the left? I do not have a clue. My interpretation is that when stutterers are more dysfluent they have a tendency, for whatever the reason, to activate the right hemisphere which then interrupts or interferes with, not only motor speech but with the perception of language in general. I think the data will bear that out. Stutterers do not have just a problem with motor speech dimensions but they do have a linguistic involvement. What we observe as part of the process is only part of the process. This is a pretty orderly disorder. Close observation indicates or supports the inference that it has a lot to do with the utilization of less effective processing strategies to process language and to use motor speech.

M. Neilson: There was a P.S. to that question which I think needs a very brief comment. Would you imagine that it would make any difference whether the fluent speech, if you test and look at hemispheric activation on fluent speech as against dysfluent speech, is achieved with the active use of fluency skills, be it whatever program, or whether it is natural fluency, a fluent run of spontaneous speech? Would you expect to see differences in the activation patterns?

W. Moore: The question is whether natural fluency in stutterers is different than artificial fluency in stutterers, in terms of the hemispheric activation patterns. I think you will find a difference in processing. I think that an artificially fluent stutterer will look like a stutterer, if he is in a "cognitive mode" to stutter. However, when normally fluent speech is used he will look like a normally fluent individual. I think that some of the procedures and strategies that we have used for years keep stutterers stuttering, fluently. Do you call *these kinds of things* (spoken at a prolonged rate) normal fluency? They are adaptive but are *vastly different than this* (spoken at normal rate). Are they functional? I think so. But, would I do it? You are darn right. I would stand right in line and do it. I think that if the stutterer is in a stuttering cognitive mode then there will be a vast difference.

H. Luper: One of the questions that came earlier from our group was one that urged you to try and see if you could separate whether or not emotions affect right hemispheric activity versus some other kinds of things. I guess I go back to that question. Could it be that if the stutterer is feeling more emotional about speech, that increased right hemispheric activity is really a sign of increased emotions about speech during stuttering?

W. Moore: I guess it could. Let us look at it in another way. Suppose the right hemisphere is importantly involved in dealing with a motive aspect of behavior and language, involved with the suprasegmental aspects which convey lots of meaning and is involved in dealing with recognition of faces and visual, spatial patterns. If now you say to the right hemisphere, "I want you not only to deal with that but I also want you to deal with some of the motor aspects of language," I think that the overload on that hemisphere, for lack of a better term, will cause an even greater problem to the stutterer. I think the environment can definitely superimpose its influence upon the stutterer in that regard. Do I think that our results are an artifact of greater right hemispheric processing because the stutterer is more emotionally involved with it? Many investigations that we have done have not asked the stutterer to do too much.

Questions from the floor

A. Caruso: I would just like to encourage you, in spite of all the problems of working with children who stutter, to really try to approach that avenue of research. I think there would be wide agreement, here and elsewhere, that this is a disorder of child-hood. I am not too sure how much of the adult data can be extracted and applied to children?

W. Moore: Okay, that is good. I do not want to make any precon-ceived speculation on it without empirical data but I want to point out that there are some studies that have been done with stutterers but not a lot. I do not want to get on yet another bandwagon that is going no place, and take the adult data and apply it to child stutterers. There may be a foundation on which we can begin to design some investigations with children.

A. Caruso: I am fascinated by the correlation that you are reporting between severity and the data you are presenting. In the speech production work I have been involved with I would be hard-pressed to come up with a similar sort of strong correlation between any index of stuttering behaviour in cinematic or EMG analysis during speech fluency or stuttered moments. I was wondering if you could address that a little more specifically. Would you include the measures of stuttering behaviour that you used, those that correlated highly, so that those of us who are trying to look again into the production data might use the same sorts of measures to see if we are getting some of the same correlations?

W. Moore: We did report those data based upon diagnostic work-ups that were done with those stutterers on spontaneous and read-ing tasks. As I recall, without getting back into the article, it was not the reading stuff that came up with the correlation. It was the spontaneous stuff that seemed to be more significantly related to the hemispheric processing. There were some conver-sations and standard passages that were read, probably the Rainbow passage. These days we use the procedure that has been recommended by BEAMS and go through all of those data. It takes hours and hours to deal with it. Those relation-ships did not pop up in the latter investigations. Now, we are concerned about levels of dysfluency in the subjects that we used in this latter investigation, in terms of why they did not come up. It seems we used fewer of your stutterers in the last two investigations. That may have had something to do with it. I do not want you to think for a moment that it is an open and shut case. It is not. What we have found, we have found. What we have not found, we have not found. There is a lot to be done in that area. You certainly know that. You deal with motor aspects of stuttering. Our results are encouraging to us.

A. Meltzer: I am very interested in the very strong statement that you made about one method of treatment being successful and another method being unsuccessful. I regularly work on both programs; those directed to modifications of speech using prolongation methods and those programs working towards normalcy of speech. I also work on programs involving both methods. I would be very interested to know what reliable good studies, and I emphasize the word reliable, there are to demonstrate that one method is superior to another in long-term maintenance.

W. Moore: I do not think I said that one was superior to another. I gave you some inferences from what I thought about those procedures and what they might be doing. I shared with you some of my conceptualizations on that. I would not even think about the studies that have looked at the difference. My concern is they have not done that. My concern is that those procedures are directly related to different neurophysiology. Many stutterers I have interacted with say "I do not like prolongation, etc. It is something that I just do not like." My clinical experience with stutterers in the last number of years has been less than it was in the past, by choice not by chance. So there is no intent of saying that this is a better procedure and that is not a better procedure.

My concern is whether we are playing into the cognitive problem of stutterers by using procedures that allow them to continue to use a less efficient or effective processing mode to gain some degree of artificial fluency. Maybe we are contributing to the problem itself. What we need to do then, is to get to an understanding of the process of which stuttering is the outcome. Certainly, simply looking at the behaviour, in and of itself, is not going to get us there. We have done that for a long time. So I am going to deal with that behaviour and I am going to make some other inferences about neurophysiology. Those are the kinds of questions that we certainly need to deal with. That is one of the questions that was asked here; "what kind of therapeutic procedures were used with those stutterers?" I think that is an important question. That is another thing that adds variance to the data. If we knew the kind of procedures that were used and we could look at them systematically, that might help us to understand what is going on. Let me underscore: *it is not my intent to say that one procedure is better than another.* There are some procedures that I just would not use out of hand; there are some procedures that I do use. If it is functional I think it is great. I think though, that we have to stop playing the game of—"Is it functional then I will go ahead and use it. I will be eclectic and I will be a wonderful stuttering therapist." I think that as a profession we need to come to grips with some deeper issues, not only in stuttering but child language and adult language disorders. I think that we delineated ourselves in the 1940s and 1950s. That was all political. It was what was happening politically at the time. It happened in psychology, spilled over into our profession and most other professions. I think that the political influence restricted what we found out about stuttering in some very important areas: neurophysiology and electrophysiology in general. We looked only at the outcome of the process.

William G. Webster

3   **Hurried Hands
and Tangled Tongues**
Implications of Current Research for
the Management of Stuttering

During the past decade I have been engaged in a
program of basic research concerned with understanding, through
an analysis of rapid hand and finger movements, some of the neural
mechanisms of stuttering, the disorder of the "tangled tongue"
(Carlisle, 1985). The research findings and ideas that have emerged
from that research appear to have implications for the clinical management of stuttering.

The origin of my interest in stuttering as a research problem lies in
my experiences as a person who stutters, and my approach to that
research problem has been influenced by my background as a
research psychologist.

I am, to use Einer Boberg's delightful expression, a "garden variety" person who stutters in that my experiences are fairly typical of
stutterers as a group: I have stuttered since I first started to talk; I
started to talk late; and there are others in my family who stutter. I
have experienced all the usual difficulties of growing up with a stutter: embarrassment, humiliation, frustration, anger, apprehension,
avoidances, and withdrawal. And, like other garden variety people
who stutter, I have found that the severity of my stuttering has varied enormously. There have been situations and periods of time
when my fluency was very good, and other situations and periods of
time when I simply could not begin to express an idea coherently.

An Overview of the Approach

One of the more striking and distinctive features of the mammalian brain is that the forebrain is comprised of two hemispheres. In the human brain, the hemispheres are so large that they obscure most of the rest of the brain except for some brainstem viewed from the ventral or lower surface. Although the two hemispheres are roughly the same size and have similar patterns of gyri and fissures which are formed by the infolding of cerebral cortex, in fact the hemispheres differ in a number of respects anatomically (Galaburda, LeMay, Kemper and Geschwind, 1978; Geschwind and Levitsky, 1968; Wada, Clarke and Hamm, 1975), neurochemically (Oke, Keller, Mefford and Adams, 1978), and functionally (Bradshaw and Nettleton, 1981; Corballis, 1983; Springer, 1986). Some of these asymmetries are alluded to by Dr. Mateer in Chapter 1. Although it is part of popular psychology to talk about right brain function and left brain function, the two hemispheres do work closely together. Their activities are coordinated through the brainstem and the various forebrain commissures like the corpus callosum and anterior commissure. In a midsaggital section of the brain, the callosum is clearly evident as a broad band of white matter comprised of an estimated 200–250 million axons (Doty and Negrao, 1973; Garey, 1979) which originate in one hemisphere and terminate in the other.

The idea that stuttering reflects a peculiarity in the relationship between the hemispheres is not new. It goes back at least 60 years to the theory and research of S.T. Orton (1928) and L.E. Travis (1931, 1978), although it fell into disfavour during the thirty-year period following World War II. As noted by Dr. Mateer in Chapter 1 and Dr. Moore in Chapter 2, interest in the idea was rekindled through the provocative report by Jones (1966) of four developmental stutterers with bilateral speech representation who became fluent following surgical excision of one apparent speech area. As summarized by Moore and Boberg (1987), the literature now contains a number of comparisons of stutterers with fluent speakers using a diverse range of methodologies. For example, studies of ear differences in dichotic listening tasks (Blood, 1985; Brady and Berson, 1975; Curry and Gregory, 1969; Rosenfield and Goodglass, 1980) and visual field differences in tachistoscopic half-field recognition tasks (Johannsen and Victor, 1986; Moore, 1976) have indicated unusual variability among people who stutter, but the data are contradictory. To the extent that ear or visual field preferences or superiority reflect aspects of hemispheric processing, as is usually assumed in the field (Springer, 1986), there would appear to be a peculiarity in this respect among stutterers. Moore (1984) has argued that the data in these various studies can be reconciled by considering stutterers to inappropriately and ineffectively engage right hemisphere strategies for processing meaningful linguistic information. He has interpreted in the same way the results of regional cerebral blood flow studies (Wood, Stump, McKennhan, Sheldon and Proctor, 1980) and EEG activation studies (Boberg, Yeudall, Schopflocher and Bo-Lassen, 1983; Moore, 1986; Moore and Haynes, 1980). These indicate that, in contrast to nonstutterers in whom there is typically greater EEG activation in the left than right hemisphere, stutterers demonstrate the reversed pattern of greater right hemisphere activation. Regardless of interpretation of the findings and despite their being inconsistent and contradictory, they do indicate anomalous interhemispheric relations of some form in stutterers or at least in a subgroup of stutterers.

As I read the literature, I found there was not a good explanation of the nature of the anomaly, nor a satisfactory understanding of possible mechanisms of stuttering, nor an understanding of how neurotransmitter function, which is known to be affected by carbohydrate consumption (e.g., Fernstrom and Wurtman, 1971), might affect those mechanisms and hence fluency. There are a number of assumptions that underlie my own research on these issues.

The *first assumption* is that there is a biological basis to stuttering. Although stuttering is clearly sex-linked, occurring more frequently in males than females (Bloodstein, 1981), it is universal in the sense that it is found in all cultures and languages (Bloodstein, 1981), and runs in families (Kidd, 1984; Sheehan and Costley, 1977), the clearest evidence for a biological or organic basis to the disorder is the results of studies involving twins. In an exceptionally well controlled study of twins, Howie (1981) reported concordance rates for stuttering of 0.73 and 0.32 for monozygotic and dizygotic twins, respectively. That the concordance for MZ twins was not 1.00 illustrates that environment and experience must in principle play a role in phenotype expression, although key factors have proved elusive to identify (Cox, Seider and Kidd, 1984).

The *second assumption* is that the particular kind of biological or organic basis of stuttering is neurological. In other words, I assume that what makes the person who stutters different in a fundamental sense from the person who does not stutter is to be found in some aspect of brain function. I assume further that variation in stuttering severity within an individual reflects variation in an aspect of brain function that relates to speech motor control.

Historically there have been two polar opposing views about the origins of stuttering and the relationship of physiological to psychological aspects of the phenomenon. At one extreme is the position that stuttering reflects a psychological or emotional disturbance. From this perspective, whatever physiological concomitants there may be are consequences of the psychological disturbance. At the other extreme is the position that stuttering reflects a physiological or neurological anomaly. From this second perspective, whatever emotional or psychological concomitants there may be are consequences and not the cause of the stuttering. My work assumes the second viewpoint. Although the primary problem in stuttering is seen to be a neurological anomaly, with emotional and psychological processes being secondary, these emotional and psychological factors clearly impact directly on the neurological anomaly and influence stuttering severity and its variability. Although emotions may be secondary, they nonetheless play an important role in the neuropsychology of stuttering.

The *third assumption*, probably the most foreign to many speech-language therapists, is that we can learn about brain mechanisms associated with speech motor control through the study of the control of other motoric processes. This idea, represented in Figure 3.1, is based on the evidence that the neural mechanisms of speech overlap the neural mechanisms involved in the control of other highly coordinated and sequential nonspeech motor processes.

Figure 3.1   A schematic representation of the idea that the brain mechanisms mediating speech and language functions overlap those mediating nonspeech motor processes.

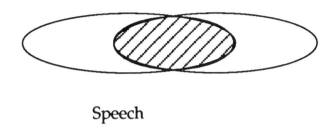

Speech

Manual Movement

The evidence for such overlap is reviewed by Mateer in Chapter 1 and in her 1983 publication. For example, the work of Doreen Kimura and her colleagues at Western Ontario (Kimura, 1977; Kimura and Archibald, 1974; Mateer and Kimura, 1977) on patients with left hemisphere brain damage indicates motor control losses both in speech and nonspeech realms. Kimura (1979; 1982) has argued that there is a common underlying mechanism that mediates these losses. Picking up on the idea developed in the early part of the twentieth century by H. Liepmann (1908), the argument has been that that the left hemisphere plays a special role in complex motor behavior, in particular with respect to the selection of individual movements and the facilitation of transitions from one movement to another. Damage to the left hemisphere interferes with these aspects of motor control regardless of whether they involve speech or nonspeech movements. It follows from these ideas that although speech and language may be one obvious dimension of brain lateralization, the more basic dimension is related to motor control (Goodale, 1988).

A second line of evidence about overlap of mechanisms is studies of electrical stimulation of exposed cerebral cortex (Ojemann, 1983;

Ojemann and Mateer, 1979; Mateer, Chap. 1). Briefly, however, electrical stimulation research has indicated that the cortex is not organized in behaviorally distinct units but instead there are many sites which when stimulated have effects on both speech and nonspeech processes.

Similar conclusions emerge from the results of studies of regional cerebral blood flow. Through tracer substances it is possible to measure blood flow in different regions of the brain (Roland, 1984). Variations in blood flow in a particular region are assumed to reflect the metabolic needs of the neurons in the region, and these needs increase with increased neuronal activity. The results of such studies of one brain area in particular, the supplementary motor area (SMA), are especially germane for our present purposes. The SMA is located mainly on the medial walls of the hemispheres just anterior to the central sulcus and above the primary motor cortex. SMA blood flow, and by implication its neural activity, increases in association both with speech or intended speech, and with actual or intended movements of fingers in particular sequences (Roland, 1985; Roland, Larsen, Lassen and Skinhoj, 1980). This is an excellent example of a brain area where mechanisms for speech overlap functionally with those for nonspeech motor control. It is an area we return to later in the context of brain mechanisms involved in stuttering.

In summary, a number of lines of evidence indicate an overlap of mechanisms. This forms the basis for adoption of an indirect approach that involves the study of nonspeech hand movements in people who stutter. What is of interest is not hand movements per se, but what those hand movements tell us about the mechanisms of speech motor control in people who stutter.

Studies of Unimanual Finger Tapping

The theoretical starting point for my research goes back a half century to the idea of Orton (1928) and Travis (1931) that there is an anomaly in interhemispheric relations associated with stuttering. The upper part of Figure 3.2 summarizes the essential features of

Figure 3.2   Two conceptualizations of anomalous interhemispheric relations in stutterers. *Upper:* A schematic representation of the model of stuttering proposed by Orton (1928) and Travis (1931). *Lower:* A schematic representation of the Interhemispheric Interference Model proposed by
Webster (1986b).

Conceptual Models

A. Orton-Travis Model

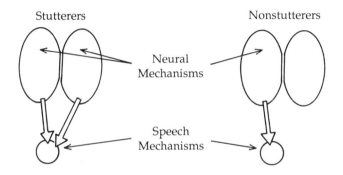

B. Interhemispheric Interference Model

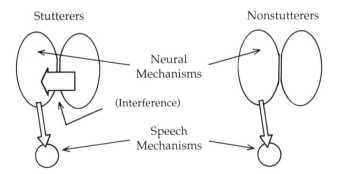

their model. It holds that the neural mechanisms mediating speech and language in stutterers are represented bilaterally rather than unilaterally in the left hemisphere. As a result, there are dual commands innervating the speech musculature. On occasion these commands are out of synchrony with one another. A consequence of such asynchrony is that the precisely timed coordination pattern of the speech musculature is disrupted, the result of which are the blockages, hesitations, and speech repetitions that constitute stuttering.

Although this is an old model, I adopted it as a starting point for my research and it has led to two very basic questions. First, could I find any evidence to support the idea that the sequencing and speech motor control mechanisms in people who stutter are represented bilaterally? A second question, influenced by characterizations of stuttering by Sheehan (1970) and Van Riper (1971), was whether I could find evidence that stuttering reflects a general problem in motor coordination, particularly when sequential responding is required?

The approach I took to these two questions was to study the ability of people who stutter to tap their fingers in particular sequences as quickly and accurately as possible. Most neurologically normal children and adults finger tap faster with the right than left hand (Denckla, 1973; Peters, 1980; Todor and Kyprie, 1980). This is often interpreted in terms of the right hand having direct access to the left hemisphere mechanisms of movement sequencing and transitions referred to earlier (Kinsbourne and McMurray, 1975; Peters, 1980; Wolff, Hurwitz and Moss, 1977). If stutterers in fact have bilateral speech mechanisms, as hypothesized by Orton (1928) and Travis (1931), and if those mechanisms overlap the nonspeech motor sequencing mechanisms, then stutterers would be expected *not to show* a right hand advantage in sequential finger tapping. Similarly, if stutterers have some general problem in motor coordination or sequencing, it should be evident in slow rates of sequential finger tapping relative to those of nonstutterer controls.

The apparatus we used to test these ideas was based on that described by Lomas and Kimura (1976). Four telegraph keys mounted in a box were each connected to a separate channel of a chart recorder so that whenever a key was pressed, it produced a pen deflection. The operation of the recorder was controlled by an interval timer. The timer was initiated by the first key press and, at the end of 15 seconds, a tone sounded to indicate the end of the trial and no further key presses were recorded.

Testing was carried out with 5 different sequences, and each subject tapped each sequence repeatedly as quickly as possible for 15 second trials with each hand. Examples of the sequences are 1–2–3–4 or 3–1–2–4 where 1 represents the index finger and 4 the little finger (the keys and fingers were never referred to by numbers when being described to the subjects). The dependent measures were the number of correct sequences tapped, incorrect key presses, and total key presses (a measure of speed).

Before describing the results, a number of points should be made about the participants used in this and the other studies to be described in this chapter. Research participants, both stutterers and nonstutterers, were recruited from the university and general community through newspaper advertisements, posters placed in the university and public places, word of mouth, media publicity, and the Stuttering Treatment Program offered at the Ottawa Rehabilitation Centre. Their ages ranged from about 16 to 55 years, with the vast majority being in the age range of 20 to 30 years. To the extent possible, control subjects were selected so their age distribution would be as similar as possible to that of the stutterers. Some studies included both right- and left-handers, operationally defined by scores on the Edinburgh Handedness Inventory (Oldfield, 1971), but other studies were restricted to right-handers. Similarly, in some studies both males and females were tested, but in others, depending on the availability of subjects, only males were used. The participants had variable treatment histories, some having never been treated and others having received many different types of treatment over many years. Reflecting the influence of Perkins (1985), the operational definition of being a stutterer was simply self-classification, as it was for the variable of sex. Severity of stuttering was assessed through self-rating scales. Subjects indicated on 7-point scales ranging from *mild* to *very severe* how severe they regarded their stuttering to be, and how severe they believed their family and friends regarded their stuttering to be. All subjects were screened for any history of neurological or movement problems and, in the case of finger tapping studies, accomplished musicians and people who earned their living by typing or keyboarding were excluded. In most studies, at least 16 stutterers and 16 nonstutterer controls were included in each major experimental condition.

This first study of repetitive sequential finger tapping (Webster, 1985) included 16 right-handed male stutterers and 16 comparable nonstutterer controls. The results which were subsequently replicated (Webster, 1986a) were clear-cut. First, a right-hand advantage for sequential finger tapping was found for both the stutterers and nonstutterers. This provided no evidence that the underlying neural mechanisms of sequential motor performance, and so by implication speech, are different in stutterers than in nonstutterers. Second, the overall performance level in terms of correct sequences and total key presses was the same in the two groups, indicating that stutterers are not generally slower motorically or more poorly coordinated.

The stutterers did make significantly more incorrect key presses than the nonstutterers although in absolute numbers these were few and had little detectable impact on the correct sequences measure. Together with the observation that two stutterers had to be excluded because they simply could not do the task, the incorrect key press data nonetheless raised questions about task sensitivity. Another concern was that all the sequences were tapped repeatedly. This is very different from the case of speech in which utterances are generally new or unique, not repeated. Furthermore, we know from the adaptation effect (Bloodstein, 1981) that fluency difficulties diminish as a phrase is repeated over and over again, and possibly finger tapping sequencing difficulties similarly had diminished with repetition.

Accordingly a new experiment (Webster, 1986a) was devised with task and motor demands that would, it was hoped, more closely approximate those of speech. Instead of having subjects repeatedly tap the same sequence over and over again, a new sequence was presented on each trial.

The apparatus was similar to that used in the first study, but there was a visual display panel which at the start of each trial indicated the particular sequence to be tapped. The panel had line drawings of the two hands, and at the end of each finger was a light emitting diode (LED), the illumination of which was controlled by a programmable microprocessor unit. To introduce unpredictability to the task, the sequences to be tapped included ones with 3 elements (e.g., 2–3–1), 4 elements (e.g., 1–3–4–3), and 5 elements (e.g., 1–2–4–2–3), but only 4-element sequences were analyzed. Some 4-element sequences contained repeated elements (e.g., 1–3–4–3) and others only unique elements (e.g., 2–1–3–4). Immediately after each sequence was presented, a tone sounded and the subject had to tap the sequence as quickly as possible for 5 seconds. In addition to analyzing the finger tapping itself, two measures of response speed were included: Response initiation time, the time that elapsed from the tone to the first key press, and response execution time, the time from the first to the fifth key press (one complete 4-element sequence).

There were three noteworthy findings. First, the stutterers made more errors and achieved fewer correct sequences than the nonstutterers. This relatively poor performance was not due to faster speed, because the stutterers were in fact significantly slower than the nonstutterers to initiate their responding. Once responding was initiated, however, the groups did not differ in response speed. The mean time required to execute the first complete sequence (when correct) was the same for the two groups, as was the mean total key presses.

One issue that concerned us was whether the sequencing problems might relate to the speeded demands of the task, and so we repeated parts of the sequence reproduction procedure under non-speeded conditions (Webster, 1989b). Subjects were told to take as much time as needed before initiating their responding to ensure accuracy. Not unexpectedly there were vast individual differences in response initiation times, and there were no overall time differences between the stutterers and nonstutterers. Nonetheless, the stutterers still made significantly more sequencing errors than the nonstutterers. In other words, removing the speeded response component did not totally ameliorate the problem. Stutterers still were less accurate than nonstutterers in reproducing the sequences.

When the data from these unimanual finger tapping studies are compared, three major points emerge. First, we have found no evidence that the neural mechanisms for motor sequencing, and by implication those of speech, are bilaterally represented as in the Orton/Travis model. The consistent right hand finger tapping advantage in stutterers and nonstutterers points instead to normal left hemisphere lateralization. This conclusion is consistent with our research on handedness distributions. We have found no evidence of greater incidence of left-handedness in stutterers nor reduced strength of handedness among right-handed stutterers (Webster and Poulos, 1987). A second point is that the person who stutters is not generally slower and/or more poorly coordinated than the nonstutterer. When the same sequence is repeatedly tapped, or once performance has been initiated on the sequence reproduction task, tapping by stutterers is as fast as by nonstutterers. The third point is that people who stutter have difficulty not only with the initiation of their speech utterances but also with nonspeech sequential motor processes. This difficulty appears to be related to response planning, organization, and initiation, and simply slowing down by itself does not ameliorate the difficulty.

Although the basic neural mechanisms of sequencing and speech in stutterers may be lateralized in the left hemisphere as they are in nonstutterers, the system does not work as efficiently and as effectively as it does in nonstutterers. Evidence of this inefficiency was seen in the errors that occasionally slipped into the repetitive finger tapping of stutterers. Clearer evidence was the difficulty of stutterers in rapidly and accurately reproducing sequences that was not ameliorated by slowing down. And of course, the idea of an inherent inefficiency is also evident in the instability of fluent speech of people who stutter (Zimmerman, 1980).

But postulating an inefficient left hemisphere system is not terribly satisfying because stuttering is not constant or stable as it might be with a brain lesion. Stuttering is highly variable and dynamic. It characteristically shows short- and long-term variation in severity, is sensitive to stress and anxiety, and is sensitive to context. And so this led to the next question: Are there other processes that could underlie the sequencing difficulties and stuttering, processes that may be involved in its variability?

Interhemispheric Interactions in Stutterers

Another possible form of anomalous interhemispheric relations can be related to how the two hemispheres interact with one another.

The lower part of Figure 3.2 reflects the thinking behind what we have called the Interhemispheric Interference Model (Webster, 1986b). Under this model, speech mechanisms are assumed to be normally lateralized in the left hemisphere as in fluent speakers. The mechanisms may not be as efficient and effective as they should be, but they are nonetheless lateralized normally. These left hemisphere mechanisms are subject to interference from activity of the right hemisphere. In other words, there may be excessive cross-talk between the hemispheres, and this cross-talk results in neural interference with the sequencing mechanisms. This is what underlies stuttering. Imagine activity in the right hemisphere "slopping over" and interfering with processing by the left hemisphere. The possible origin and nature of the cross-talk and interference are discussed later.

One obvious and direct way to test this idea would be to cut the corpus callosum, the fibres that interconnect the hemispheres. The prediction of the model clearly is that such a procedure would reduce stuttering because of the reduction in interhemispheric interference. This type of surgery is carried out for the relief of intractable epilepsy and results in some neuropsychologically fascinating phenomena (Sperry, 1974), but there have been no reported cases of patients who stutter. A close approximation, that of partial disconnection, may be the four cases of Jones (1966) alluded to earlier. All underwent cortical excisions for the treatment of neurological conditions apparently unrelated to stuttering. Such an excision necessarily involves a partial disconnection of the hemispheres because it damages callosal fibres that have their origin or termination in the excised cortex. What is provocative is that the cortical excisions in Jones's (1966) patients were anterior and postoperatively speech fluency was reported to have improved markedly.

Testing the model does not require such invasive means as

surgery. There are a number of indirect methods available from neu-ropsychology. These involve variations on the children's game of rubbing your stomach and patting your head at the same time. If you have no callosum to connect the hemispheres this is a very easy task because there is no interference between the hands and they function independently (Preilowski, 1975); to the extent there is cross-talk between the hemispheres the task is made difficult by the tendency for mirror-image movements (Fog and Fog, 1963). The degree of functional linkage between the hemispheres can be assessed then through the study of the interaction between the hands. We have done this now in a number of studies with stutterers.

The first two studies of bimanual interaction followed directly from the earlier work on unimanual finger tapping. They involved an analysis of how repetitive sequential finger tapping (Webster, 1986b) and sequence reproduction performance (Webster, 1989a) by the right hand is affected by a motor activity carried out concurrently with the left hand. The concurrent task required the subject to hold and turn a knob back and forth every time a brief tone sounded. In other words, while the subject was tapping telegraph keys in particular sequences with the right hand, he had to listen for tones and respond to them with a motor movement by the left hand. The model predicts that stutterers will have greater difficulty than nonstutterers on such a dual-task, and indeed that is what was found for both types of tapping tasks. Not surprisingly, all subjects had reduced tapping performance under conditions of concurrent task testing conditions. What was of significance, however, was that the stutterers showed a greater performance decrement. It is important to stress that not only was their sequence tapping performance poorer than the nonstutterers, but the accuracy of the knob turning performance was poorer as well.

These results then are consistent with the model. When right hemisphere activity was increased through the left handed task, the interference on the left hemisphere increased as evidenced in greater decrements by stutterers than nonstutterers in right hand performance.

In a third study, I moved away from sequential finger tapping and looked at bimanual interaction that involved handwriting performance (Webster, 1988). As described earlier, there is a natural tendency for the limbs to move in a mirror-image manner (Fog and Fog, 1963). Independence of movement depends upon functional separation of the hemispheres. Split-brain cases have good independence (Preilowski, 1975); young children have poor independence (Connolly and Stratton, 1968). An implication of the interhemispheric interference model is that people who stutter should be more like young children, i.e., show a greater tendency towards mirror-image movements. When writing letters simultaneously with the two hands, the greater linkage between the hemispheres should be evident in a greater number of mirror-reversed letters written with the nonpreferred hand.

This idea was tested by having subjects write letters with the two hands simultaneously on upright writing surfaces, using an apparatus similar to the Van Riper (1934) Critical Angle Board. A cloth separated the subject from the apparatus so the hands and the writing could not be seen. Without going into much detail here on procedures, on any given trial the subject was required to write four letters with the two hands simultaneously. These were to be written as quickly as possible one under the other. Performance was timed, and a standardized system was developed whereby the letters were scored for evidence of mirror-reversed components and for overall quality. The rating was done by judges who were not aware of the identity or testing conditions of the subjects. Under the model, the stutterers were predicted to do poorly particularly with regard to mirror-reversed letters with the left hand.

The actual design of the study was complex in that it included males and females and right- and left-handers, and subjects were tested with varying angles between the writing surfaces. But the results were clear-cut. The stutterers, both males and females, took longer to write the letters than did the nonstutterers. Second, the stutterers made more mirror-reversed letters than the nonstutterers, and overall letter quality was significantly poorer. Consistent with the two dual-task studies described earlier, the results of this study make clear that there is more bimanual interference in stutterers than in nonstutterers, and we interpret this to mean more interhemispheric interference.

But this interpretation does lead to a critical question: Do the bimanual interference effects reflect *interhemispheric* processes, or do they reflect difficulty in the effective allocation of attention in simultaneous information processing? In other words, could it be that stutterers have greater difficulty than nonstutterers in doing any two tasks at the same time, not just tasks that involve different hemispheres?

This is a very open question. A graduate student in my lab, David Forster, has examined it through a study of the interaction of the hands and feet of the two sides of the body in stutterers and nonstutterers. The study involves a dual-task paradigm similar to that used by Webster (1986b) but instead of tasks being finger tapping with one hand and knob turning with the other, they are finger tapping with one hand and paced foot movements with one foot. If the hypothesized interference is limited to interhemispheric mechanisms, then stutterers should show greater interference than nonstutterers when using the hand on one side of the body and the foot on the other, but no greater interference than nonstutterers when using the hand and foot on the same side of the body. However, if the interference is of a more general nature, then the interference effects for hand-foot combinations on the same side of the body should be equivalent to those for hand-foot combinations on the opposite sides of the body. This work is still in progress and it would be premature to describe any preliminary data.

There is one study I have done, however, which does suggest the interference may be more general (Webster, 1987). The task is what we call a letter sequence transcription task, and it requires the subject on any given trial to transcribe to paper sequences of letters (such as N A S B O C R) presented aurally at a rate faster than can be written. The length of the sequences ranged from 3 to 10 letters. Accuracy of transcription was assessed in a number of ways, but the gist of the results is clear simply in the significantly lower probability by stutterers than nonstutterers of correctly transcribing sequences of all lengths including the shortest. The nature of the problem is still unclear (Webster, 1990a). Stutterers have a real problem with this task when there are dual processing components but there is no reason to think that the components are mediated by different hemispheres. This suggests some more general problem of interference regardless of whether one or both hemispheres are involved.

Another indication that the problem may relate in part to the effective allocation of attention comes from work on rhythmic finger tapping by the two hands. Peters (1987) developed a 2:1 tapping task which required subjects to tap a key twice with one hand for each single tap of a key by the other hand. He reported that right-handers (nonstutterers) perform this task better when it is the right hand that taps twice (R2/L1 condition) rather than the left hand (L2/R1 condition), but among left-handers performance is similar under the two tapping conditions. Peters has drawn upon Annett's (1978) single gene model of handedness which suggests that right-handers but not left-handers have an inherent directional bias and has argued that the differences observed between his right- and left-handers reflects the role of attention in the expression of handedness. More specifically, he has argued that right-handers have an attentional bias to the right hand that facilitates performance in the R2/L1 condition, but left-handers are more flexible in focusing lateralized attention and can attend with equal facility to the right or left hand when leading. Underlying this right side attentional bias in right-handers is thought to be a tonic left hemisphere activation, and in contrast there is a greater lability of hemispheric activation in left-handers.

Because of this attentional interpretation, I carried out a study (Webster, 1990b) of 2:1 finger tapping by stutterers using a slightly different methodology from that of Peters (1987). The design included both males and females, and of course right- and left-handers, tested under the two tapping conditions. On any given trial subjects were to tap the rhythm as quickly as possible for 10 seconds. The trial was repeated until it was performed correctly. One dependent measure was the number of attempts required for four correct trials. The second, speed of performance, was assessed by counting the number of taps by the lead hand on the four correct trials. The results were clear-cut. First, among the nonstutterers the results replicated Peters's findings: Right-handers indeed did perform better on the R2/L1 than on the L2/R1 condition, but there was no such asymmetry in left-handers. More germane to the present discussion was that the overall rate of tapping that could be achieved while being accurate was much less in stutterers than in nonstutterers. This again illustrates the interference seen in stutterers when doing two things at the same time. Second, and perhaps of more interest with respect to mechanisms, was the finding that the right-handed stutterers were similar to left-handed nonstutterers in that tapping proficiency was the same for the two tapping conditions. Following from Peters's interpretation of the performance asymmetry, the results suggested then that stutterers have a greater lability or flexibility of hemispheric activation or biasing than do nonstutterers. This of course assumes that the underlying reason for performance symmetry is the same in stutterers as in left-handed nonstutterers.

These research findings on bimanual performance by stutterers lead to the general conclusion that stuttering is not a speech disorder as such, although speech is one obvious and prominent manifestation. Instead, stuttering reflects anomalous information processing that is evident in nonspeech motor and cognitive activities. More specifically, the anomalies associated with stuttering appear to be related to response planning, organization, and initiation, and possibly to attentional mechanisms. But what is the nature of the anomaly?

A Working Model of Brain Mechanisms and Stuttering

The research on unimanual and bimanual motor performance in stutterers has led to and is driven by a working model of brain mechanisms underlying stuttering that has three major elements:

1. The neural mechanisms for speech and sequencing processes in stutterers are lateralized normally in the left hemisphere.
2. These left hemisphere neural mechanisms for sequencing and speech in stutterers are "fragile" and susceptible to interference from other on-going neural activities.
3. There is a labile or unstable pattern of hemispheric activation in stutterers.

The first element of the model is based on our consistent findings of the same right hand advantage in stutterers as found in nonstutterers for unimanual motor control.

The second element of the model has two parts. First, what I mean by the system being "fragile" is that it does not operate as efficiently or as effectively as it should due to some underlying structural and functional problem with the circuitry. The evidence for such inefficiency was reviewed earlier. The second part is the idea of interference, and this is based on the results of the several dual-task experiments we have carried out. This susceptibility to disruption by other neural processes may simply be one aspect of the inefficiency or fragility of the system.

The third element of the model, lability of hemispheric activation, is derived from our interpretation of the results of the 2:1 tapping study. To some extent as well it is based on the findings of Boberg et al. (1983) and Moore (1986) of unusual right hemisphere activation in stutterers.

The Supplementary Motor Area as a Locus for Interference

A first issue that arises in considering this working model is just where the fragile system is supposed to be located or where the hypothesized interference is supposed to take place. My working hypothesis at this time is that it is useful to look at the supplementary motor area (SMA).

Because of its location, the SMA has been difficult to study both in human patients and experimental animals, but there is a growing body of literature concerning its functions. Much of this literature has been reviewed by Wise (1984), Goldberg (1985), and Wiesendanger (1986). At the risk of oversimplification, the frontal cortex can be anatomically and functionally divided into the granular or prefrontal cortex, occupying the anterior part of the hemispheres, and the agranular or precentral cortex lying between the central sulcus and prefrontal cortex. This precentral cortex can be divided into primary motor cortex, the electrical stimulation of which results in discrete body movements, and nonprimary premotor cortex, which appears to be more involved in the planning and organization of movement. SMA and premotor cortex are related but discrete components of the nonprimary motor cortex. SMA receives extensive inputs from the superior parietal lobule and the basal ganglia, and has major connections to the motor cortex and cerebellum. Of special relevance to the present discussion, SMA has very rich interhemispheric connections through the corpus callosum. All cortically mediated interhemispheric interactions of the motor system are through SMA. In a meaningful sense, then, SMA is a central and key part of the motor control system.

Since the area was first identified by Penfield and Welch (1949; 1951), SMA structure and function have been studied using a number of methodologies. A sense of its importance in motor organization can be derived by considering simply three rather representative sets of findings. First, regional cerebral blood flow studies (Roland, 1985) indicate this area becomes active during actual or intended speech and during actual or intended sequential manual movement. What appears to be important is not movement per se, but the planning and organization of movements involving sequences. Second, neuropsychological analysis of patients with damage to the SMA points to a role also in response initiation. Such patients are often mute for a period following damage, and after speech recovers they typically continue to have difficulty initiating speech and engage in little spontaneous speech (Jonas, 1981). An analogous form of apraxia for transitive limb movements has been reported for patients with similar damage (Watson, Fleet, Gonzalez-Rothi and Heilman, 1986). A third set of findings comes from neurophysiology. Studies of single cell activity in experimental animals (Tanji, Taniguchi and Suga, 1980) and of slow wave potentials in intact human subjects (Deecke, Kornhuber, Lang, Lang and Schreiber, 1985; Kornhuber and Deecke, 1965) have reported electrophysiological changes in SMA that become evident long before any actual overt movement occurs.

This kind of evidence has led to the view that the SMA is critically involved not so much in the execution of movement as in its planning, control, and initiation (Goldberg, 1985; Wiesendanger, 1986). Accordingly it should not be surprising that I have proposed (Webster, 1988) this area to be a prime candidate as the locus of a problem in people who stutter. There are a number of lines of evidence to support this idea.

First, the difficulties encountered by people who stutter on various kinds of manual performance tasks parallel those they encounter in speech. This suggests that wherever and whatever the problem in the nervous system that underlies stuttering, it involves an area where there is overlap between speech and nonspeech motoric processes. The SMA is one obvious site of such overlap.

Second, the difficulties of stutterers appear to relate to motor planning and initiation of new sequences of movements, and, the integrity of the SMA appears critical for these processes.

Third, the bimanual handwriting study suggested some form of overflow between the hemispheres, and again this points to supplementary motor area as a mediator. It is through SMA that the motor systems of the two hemispheres are interconnected; it is not through primary motor cortex. Furthermore, research with nonhuman primates (Brinkman, 1984) has indicated that SMA damage results in a loss of bimanual coordination due to the release of mirror-image movements by the two hands, a condition that is resolved following disconnection of the hemispheres by callosectomy.

It is not only my research program and theorizing that has implicated SMA. Caruso, Abbs and Gracco (1988) reached a similar conclusion on the basis of their elegant studies of the coordination of lip and jaw movements of stutterers. Similarly using imaging and evoked potential methods, Pool, Freeman and Finitzo (1987) have reported similar indications of a critical SMA role in both spasmodic dysphonia and stuttering.

In summary, I see the supplementary motor area to be one possible candidate for where the fragile part of the system may be located and for where the interference that I talk about may be taking place.

The Origin or Nature of the Interference

Before considering the origin or nature of interference, we should remind ourselves of four principles of cortical organization.

The first principle is the *modular organization* of the cerebral cortex. The cells of the cerebral cortex are not simply distributed as a large homogeneous mass, but they are instead organized into columns which are thought to comprise functional modules of the cortex (Goldman-Rakic, 1984; Mountcastle, 1978).

A second principle, based on the study of sensory cortex but thought to apply equally to all areas of cortex (Cook, 1986), is that adjacent columns inhibit one another. The significance of this process of *reciprocal* or *lateral inhibition* probably is that it serves to enhance the functional differentiation of cortical modules. In other words, pericolumnar inhibition serves to increase the difference between those modules that are involved at a given instant in processing and those that should not be active at that instant.

A third principle is that columns of one hemisphere are connected through the callosum or anterior commissure to those of the other hemisphere. This point-to-point type of projection is called *homotopic*, and the evidence for it has been well reviewed by Cook (1986).

A fourth principle is that the columns of the cortex receive inputs not only from other cortical sites in the same and opposite hemisphere, but there is also a tonic activation of the columns through brainstem mechanisms. When we are talking about hemispheric activation, in some measure at least we are talking about the results of such input from the brainstem.

Following from these four principles are a number of possible hypotheses one could reasonably entertain about the nature of the interference operating on the structurally fragile left supplementary motor area in stutterers. The possibilities range from ones of local or molecular nature to ones that are far more global. The three I will discuss briefly cover that range.

One possible mechanism of inefficiency and/or interference operating at a local or molecular level relates to *pericolumnar inhibition*. If the columns do not inhibit one another sufficiently, as might be the case if there were a deficiency of some transmitter substance or if the inhibitory neurons were not sufficiently myelinated, one could imagine interference in behavior resulting from nonfocused cortical activity. It was suggested earlier that reciprocal inhibition among cortical columns is a mechanism to enhance functional differentiation. As the level of activity in one column is increased, the level of activity in the adjacent columns which may mediate potentially competing or conflicting movements is decreased. With complex, highly coordinated, and precisely timed movements, one would imagine performance enhancement with such functional differentiation. Precision and crispness on the output undoubtedly requires corresponding precision and crispness in the mechanisms.

I know of no evidence that indicates that stutterers in fact suffer from inadequate pericolumnar inhibition, but also I know of no attempt to test the idea (nor, indeed, of the techniques and methods one might reasonably employ to do so at this time), but I include this as a speculative possibility in this discussion for a number of reasons. First I wish to make the point that interference with neural processing could be occurring at a relatively local level. Second, the basic mechanisms that might underlie the inhibitory deficiency (e.g., transmitter substance anomalies or inadequate myelination) are ones that would be consistent with clinical observations on spontaneous remission in children. And third, this is an example of one mechanism which could underlie the inefficiency of the fragile SMA. In other words, inadequate pericolumnar inhibition is an example of what I mean by "structural weakness" of an inefficient neural system.

A second possibility of a mechanism of interference is what I have called "ungated callosal function" (Webster, 1986b). This is very much what I was referring to earlier in the context of the Interhemispheric Interference Model (Figure 3.2) that led to our dual-task experiments.

By ungated callosal function, I am referring to a very general possibility that information flow between the hemispheres is not coordinated properly. A useful analogy for thinking about this is two computers interacting through a connecting cable. For computers to communicate requires what is called a communication protocol. This specifies the precise conditions for communication and coordinates the two systems so that when one is ready to send the other is ready to receive. If that coordination is lacking, one could imagine signals from computer A interfering with current processing in computer B. It is to be noted that if the computers are not coordinated, the problem is probably not in the cable itself; it is more likely in the communication protocol programs (computer software) or in how the cable pins have been connected to the connector plugs (computer hardware). Returning to the brain, if there is a lack of coordination in interhemi-

spheric communication so that activity in one hemisphere can interfere with activity in the other, the origin of the problem is likely to be
found in the cortex. Remember that the callosum is comprised simply
of axons, and those axons originate and terminate in the cortex. This
brings us back again to think about the SMA, an area with many cells
having axons that are part of the callosum. To get really speculative,
one could imagine that if there were insufficient pericolumnar inhibition within the SMA, one manifestation might be interhemispheric
interference from over-active surrounding columns.

Still another possible source of interference, and one that is at the
global end of the continuum, is "attentional lability." Perhaps this is
similar to the idea that Dr. Moore in Chapter 2 alluded to of there
being nonfocused attention in stutterers. But what I am referring to
by this is a possible failure of frontal lobe executive function to sustain attention properly to information processing.

One conceptualization of the prefrontal cortex (Stuss and Benson,
1986) is that it functions as an executive that monitors current neural
processing through the brain and allocates time or resources to different possible activities. Part of the basis for this conceptualization
comes from the study of patients with frontal lobe damage. One
characteristic of such patients is that in unstructured and novel situations, attention is not well sustained and the person is easily dis-
tracted. The conceptualization is also based on a consideration of the
anatomical connections to and from prefrontal cortex. The prefrontal
cortex receives connections from virtually all areas of cerebral cortex
and has efferent connections to those same areas. Anatomically it is
well situated to monitor on-going sensory, cognitive, and affective
activities, and in turn to direct attention and processing resources to
selected activities.

To use again a computer analogy, time-sharing computers have
part of the system dedicated to monitoring what is going on at various terminals. They use programmed decision rules to let each termi-
nal have appropriate access to the central computing unit for an
appropriate amount of time. In terms of brain function and speech,
instead of there being sustained activity in the left hemisphere modules, perhaps the frontal control system permits or directs right hemisphere modules to become activated at the wrong times. Figure 3.3 is

Figure 3.3   A schematic representation of a labile hemispheric activation system showing shifts of attention towards and away from left hemisphere SMA processing modules. The relative size of areas and arrows represent activity levels and potential interference, respectively.

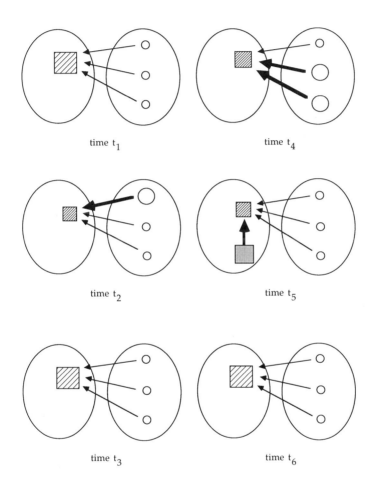

intended to illustrate this idea. At time t_1, attention is focused on the left hemisphere sequencing mechanisms. Instead of being sustained, attention shifts at time t_2 to right hemisphere modules. The effect of this shift is to reduce activation of the left hemisphere modules and to provide a source of potential interference with the remaining activity in the left hemisphere modules. Attention then shifts back to the left hemisphere modules at time t_3 but because of the lability or instability it shifts again at time t_4 to other right hemisphere modules. Just to make clear that I do not necessarily view this entirely as an interhemispheric lability, I have indicated a shift of attention at time t_5 to other left hemisphere modules before attention returns at time t_6 to the left hemisphere SMA.

Obviously there are many possibilities as to the nature of the hypothesized interference. To summarize just a few of them, perhaps the interference effects reflect just an inefficient left SMA. The structural weakness of the system may simply make it vulnerable to interference from any other on-going neural activity. Alternatively, the interference effects might reflect a problem of gating of information flow from one hemisphere to the other. Within this possibility, the SMA perhaps is not particularly vulnerable to neural activity elsewhere, it is just that it is bombarded with potentially interfering activity. Still another alternative is that the interference effects are not a gating problem but reflect an unusually high level of right hemisphere activation which overflows to the left hemisphere. There are other possibilities as well. Although at this time we cannot clearly differentiate among them, I would like to pick up on these ideas and return to the basic question with which we started: what underlies variability in stuttering? Perhaps by doing so some of my preferences, biases and hypotheses about mechanisms may become more evident.

Variability in Stuttering Severity

One feature of our working model of brain mechanisms and stuttering is the idea of a "fragile" supplementary motor area. This is what is hypothesized to underlie the basic motor control problem, the core disfluency. Another feature of the model is the idea of a labile and unstable pattern of hemispheric activation. It should be clear from my earlier comments that I see right hemisphere activation as an important source of interference with the left SMA, although probably not the only source. It follows from this that it is the labile activation that underlies stuttering severity. Factors that promote lability and hence right hemisphere activation during speech will increase neural interference on the left SMA and hence increase stuttering severity. One obvious example of such a factor is the arousal of negative emotions.

It is becoming increasingly clear that positive and negative emotions are mediated differentially by the two hemispheres (Davidson, 1984; Kinsbourne, 1982). For example, Ahern and Schwartz (1985) have found that the experience and expression of negative emotions and behavioral withdrawal is accompanied in normal fluent individuals by an EEG pattern reflecting right hemisphere activation. When these same individuals experience and express positive emotions and behavioral approach there is a left hemisphere EEG activation pattern. Davidson and Fox (1982) and Fox and Davidson (1988) have reported very similar findings with infants.

One thing that characterizes "garden variety" stutterers is negative affect and withdrawal with respect to social and speaking situations (Sheehan, 1970). And so given a fragile supplementary motor area that is closely linked to the right hemisphere through the callosum, given a labile activation system, and given a propensity for right hemisphere activation due to emotional and psychological processes, there are all the makings for a neural amplification system. As the right hemisphere becomes active due to the arousal of negative affect and withdrawal, its increased activity acts on the fragile left SMA increasing its inherent inefficiency and ineffectiveness and in turn increasing stuttering. This in turn will reinforce the negative affect and withdrawal, and correspondingly right hemisphere activation.

An implication of this line of reasoning is that the degree of baseline dysfluency in an individual reflects the nature of the structural weakness of the left SMA. By contrast, the variability that rides on top of that baseline dysfluency reflects the operation of factors that affect right hemisphere activation. I suggested negative emotions and withdrawal as an example of such a factor, but it is important to recognize that there are probably others as well, including attention to prosodic (Ross and Mesulam, 1979) and emotional (Ley and Bryden, 1982) features of speech, engagement in performance demanding high attention (Deutsch, Papanicolaou, Bourbon and Eisenberg, 1987), or depression (Schaffer and Davidson, 1983).

Implications for Stuttering Treatment and Management

I believe that this line of research on manual movement control and the ideas it has led to about brain mechanisms have implications for our understanding of stuttering treatment and for the successful management of stuttering.

In broad conceptual terms, we have come to view stuttering as resulting from a fragile speech motor control system that is vulnerable to interference. This idea is summarized schematically in Figure 3.4.

One implication of the model is that a cure or reversal of stuttering is unlikely. The key element of the model is that there is some basic mis-wiring or some missing ingredient in the "chemical soup" of the SMA. There is no reason to believe at this time that this anomaly is or can be reversed by therapy. Let me add two qualifiers. First, this strong claim relates only to *adults* who stutter. The research on which the model is based was carried out with adults, and accordingly generalizations are limited to them. It is certainly the case that adults who stutter were once children who stuttered, but there are many children who stutter who do not become adults who stutter (Andrews and Harris, 1964). The basic underlying problem in speech motor control in many young children who stutter may indeed be reversible or correctable with therapy or perhaps simply through continued maturation. Speculation was offered earlier on possible mechanisms of such reversal. One priority area for empirical research must be directed to the psychobiological differentiation of those children whose stutter-

Figure 3.4   A schematic representation of the idea of a fragile motor control system being impinged upon by sources of interference.

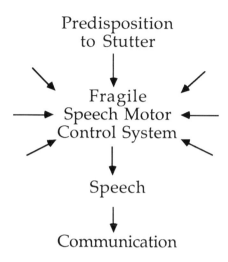

ing improves from those whose stuttering continues into adulthood. A second qualifier is that depending on the nature of the anomaly in adults, it may in fact prove to be reversible. For example, if the fragility should be related to a neurochemical imbalance, reversal may be entirely possible directly through pharmacological or dietary manipulations or indirectly through cognitive and behavioral means. However, if it should be related to something like incomplete myelination of axons, then reversal would seem more unlikely. We simply do not know, although at this time my bias is to view the anomaly in adults as being basically nonreversible.

A second implication is that successful treatment in adults has its effects by compensating for the fragility, not by reversing or correcting the underlying problem. Therapy teaches skills that lead to control.

The third implication is that control will last only as long as the compensatory skills are applied. Although the physiology of the system may be *controlled* by skills, the skills do not permanently alter that physiology, and hence the system remains inherently fragile and will revert to an unstable state if the control skills are not used.

To return to the second implication, in what sense can stuttering treatment teach skills that control the physiology of the system? At the risk of oversimplification, adult stuttering treatment has generally been of two different sorts. The first is fluency shaping, in which the emphasis is on the acquisition and use of motoric skills related to breathing, voice onset, and prolongation of sounds (e.g., R.L. Webster, 1980). The second is desensitization, in which the emphasis is on reduction of fear and avoidance (Sheehan, 1970). Note that differences in approach are largely ones of emphasis, and almost any contemporary therapy involves both elements to some extent.

For example, desensitization is often accompanied by training in voluntary controlled repetitions (VCRs) to minimize blocking. On the other hand, fluency shaping often requires work with clients to reduce fears and avoidances (Webster and Poulos, 1989).

Based on earlier comments, I think that these two components of treatment may affect fluency through fundamentally different mechanisms.

The modification of speech or stuttering, through skills like breathing control, gentle onsets, prolongations, or VCRs all involve some simplification of the speech process. They bring the production of speech into the realm of capability of the inefficient left hemisphere SMA mechanisms. I suspect as well that the deliberate, voluntary, and systematic use of these skills provides structure to the speaking situation (which helps focus attention). I also suspect that the deliberate, voluntary, and systematic use of these skills requires that the left hemisphere regain and retain control. In other words use of fluency skills or techniques emphasizes the left hemisphere mechanisms rather than testing them.

I like to think that desensitization, which is concerned with reducing negative affect and withdrawal associated with speaking situations, has its effect on right hemisphere mechanisms. By reducing fear and avoidance, right hemisphere activation is reduced and there is a more stable system. Although stable, it is not a system that leads necessarily to fluent speech because the left hemisphere mechanisms are still inefficient and are still being used beyond their capacity. But what has happened is that one important source of *potential interference* that can overflow into the structurally weak left hemisphere system has been reduced. Looking at this in another way, desensitization brings under control a mechanism that can amplify the left SMA inefficiency.

The two aspects of contemporary adult stuttering treatment are complementary and have their effects on speech control through very different brain mechanisms. Fluency shaping has the effect of compensating for an inherent inefficiency of the left hemisphere mechanisms and of enhancing left hemisphere function. Desensitization, on the other hand, has the effect of reducing right hemisphere activation associated with negative affect and withdrawal, this minimizes overflow into a structurally weak system, and that in turn keeps the inherent inefficiency or weakness from being amplified beyond some baseline level.

Let me bring this line of speculation to a close with a number of questions about treatment that arise from it. Is there an optimal way to combine fluency shaping and desensitization in treatment? Can we differentiate between severe stuttering due to hypothesized left hemisphere fragility and severe stuttering due to hypothesized right hemisphere interference effects, and can we aim treatment appropriately? In other words, are there particular types of clients defined in terms of brain mechanisms for whom one component should be stressed over the other? What outcomes can be expected realistically from treatment that emphasizes one or the other component? Does there come a time when the systematic use of fluency and desensitization skills becomes so routine and automatic that, for all practical purposes, stuttering is cured? These are but a few of many theoretically and clinically interesting questions to be explored through joint ventures of neuropsychology and speech-language pathology.

Conclusion

Stuttering is usually characterized as a speech disorder involving involuntary sound repetitions, prolongations, or hesitations (e.g.,

Andrews and Harris, 1964; Wingate, 1964). The results of the research I have described indicate that while this may be an adequate characterization for many descriptive and clinical purposes, it does not capture the underlying basis of the phenomenon. The results indicate instead that the brain of the person who stutters differs from that of the nonstutterer, and the speech disruptions associated with stuttering are just one of a number of motor and cognitive manifestations of the anomaly.

This past decade has seen the development and refinement of a number of methodologies for the study of brain function in normal and clinical populations. As we continue to apply these and develop a better understanding of the nature of the brain anomaly in people who stutter, we can expect to understand better the nature of the phenomenon of stuttering and its treatment, and to move beyond the highly speculative domain encountered in this presentation. Equally important from the point of view of a neuropsychologist is the promise that by studying in people who stutter the varied motor and cognitive manifestations of what will probably prove to be a rather minor brain anomaly we will gain insights into the normal organization and functioning of the brain as it relates to behavior.

Acknowledgments

Preparation of this chapter and the research of the author described in it were supported by a grant from the Natural Sciences and Engineering Research Council of Canada. The author expresses sincere appreciation to Joanne Hakkaku for her careful and patient testing of research participants and scoring data protocols. Without her assistance over the years the research would not have been done as well. The author also acknowledges with gratitude the invaluable benefit he has received from discussions with Marie Poulos of many of the ideas developed in this paper, particularly those that relate to clinical issues.

References

Ahern, G.L. and Schwartz, G.E. (1985). Differential lateralization for positive and negative emotion in the human brain: EEG spectral analysis. *Neuropsychologia* 23: 745–55.

Andrews, G. and Harris, M.M. (1964). *The syndrome of stuttering. Clinics in Developmental Medicine,* No. 17. London: Spastics Society Medical Education and Information Unit/Heinemann.

Annett, M. (1978). *A single gene explanation of right and left handedness and brainedness.* Coventry: Lanchester Polytechnic.

Blood, G.W. (1985). Laterality differences in child stutterers: Heterogeneity, severity levels, and statistical treatments. *Journal of Speech and Hearing Disorders* 50: 66–72.

Bloodstein, O. (1981). *A handbook of stuttering,* 3rd edition. Chicago: The National Easter Seal Society.

Boberg, E., Yeudall, L.T., Schopflocher, D. and Bo-Lassen, P. (1983). The effect of an intensive behavioral program on the distribution of EEG alpha power in stutterers during the processing of verbal and visuospatial information. *Journal of Fluency Disorders* 8: 245–63.

Bradshaw, J.L. and Nettleton, N.C. (1981). The nature of hemispheric specialization in man. *The Behavioral and Brain Sciences* 4: 51–91.

Brady, J.P. and Berson, J. (1975). Stuttering, dichotic listening, and cerebral dominance. *Archives of General Psychiatry* 32: 1449–52.

Brinkman, C. (1984). Supplementary motor area of the monkey's cerebral cortex: Short- and long-term deficits after unilateral ablation and the effects of subsequent callosal section. *Journal of Neuroscience* 4: 918–29.

Carlisle, J.A. (1985). *Tangled tongue: Living with a stutter.* Toronto: University of Toronto Press.

Caruso, A.J., Abbs, J.H. and Gracco, V.L. (1988). Kinematic analysis of multiple movement coordination during speech in stutterers. *Brain* 111: 439–55.

Connolly, K. and Stratton, P. (1968). Developmental changes in associated movements. *Developmental Medicine and Child Neurology* 10: 49–56.

Cook, N.D. (1986). *The brain code.* London: Methuen.

Cox, N.J., Seider, R.A. and Kidd, K.K. (1984). Some environmental factors and hypotheses for stuttering in families with several stutterers. *Journal of Speech and Hearing Research* 27: 543–48.

Corballis, M.C. (1983). *Human laterality.* New York: Academic Press.

Curry, F.K.W. and Gregory, H.H. (1969). The performance of stutterers on dichotic listening tasks thought to reflect cerebral dominance. *Journal of Speech and Hearing Research* 12: 73–82.

Davidson, R.J. (1984). Hemispheric asymmetry and emotion. In K.R. Scherer and P. Ekman, eds., *Approaches to emotion*. Hillsdale, NJ: Erlbaum.

Davidson, R.J. and Fox, N.A. (1982). Asymmetrical brain activity discriminates between positive versus negative affective stimuli in ten month old infants. *Science* 218: 1235–37.

Deecke, L. and Kornhuber, H.H. (1978). An electrical sign of participation of the mesial "supplementary" motor cortex in human voluntary finger movement. *Brain Research* 159: 473–76.

Deecke, L., Kornhuber, H.H., Lang, W., Lang, M. and Schreiber, H. (1985). Timing function of the frontal cortex in sequential motor and learning tasks. *Human Neurobiology* 4: 143–54.

Denckla, M.B. (1973). Development of speed in repetitive and successive finger-movements in normal children. *Developmental Medicine and Child Neurology* 15: 635–45.

Deutsch, G., Papanicolaou, A.C., Bourbon, W.T., and Eisenberg, H.M. (1987). Cerebral blood flow evidence of right frontal activation in attention demanding tasks. *International Journal of Neuropsychology* 36: 23–28.

Doty, R.W. and Negrao, N. (1973). Forebrain commissures and vision. In R. Jung, ed., *Handbook of Sensory Physiology*, Vol. VII/3B, pp. 543-82. Berlin: Springer.

Fernstrom, J.D. and Wurtman, R.J. (1971). Brain serotonin content: Increase following ingestion of carbohydrate diet. *Science* 174: 1023–25.

Fog, E. and Fog, M. (1963). Cerebral inhibition examined by associated movements. In M. Bax and R.C. MacKeith, eds., *Minimal cerebral dysfunction*, pp. 52–57. London: Spastics Society Medical Education and Information Unit/Heinemann.

Fox, N.A. and Davidson, R.J. (1988). Patterns of brain electrical activity during facial signs of emotion in 10-month-old infants. *Developmental Psychology* 24: 230–36.

Galaburda, A.M., LeMay, M., Kemper, T.L. and Geschwind, N. (1978). Right-left asymmetries in the brain. *Science* 199: 852–56.

Garey, L.J. (1979). Mammalian neocortical commissures. In I.S. Russell et al., eds., *Structure and function of the cerebral commissures*, pp. 147–54. New York: Macmillan.

Geschwind, N. and Levitsky, W. (1968). Human brain: Left-right asymmetries in temporal speech region. *Science* 16: 186–87.

Goldberg, G. (1985). Supplementary motor area structure and function: Review and hypotheses. *The Behavioral and Brain Sciences* 8: 567–616.

Goldman-Rakic, P.S. (1984). Modular organization of prefrontal cortex. *Trends in Neurosciences* 7: 419–24.

Goodale, M.A. (1988). Hemispheric differences in motor control. *Behavioural Brain Research* 30: 203–14.

Howie, P.M. (1981). Concordance for stuttering in monozygotic and dizygotic twin pairs. *Journal of Speech and Hearing Research* 24: 317–21.

Johannsen, H.S. and Victor, C. (1986). Visual information processing in the left and right hemispheres during unilateral tachistoscopic stimulation of stutterers. *Journal of Fluency Disorders* 11: 285–91.

Jonas, S. (1981). The supplementary motor region and speech emission. *Journal of Communication Disorders* 14: 349–73.

Jones, R.K. (1966). Observations on stammering after localized cerebral injury. *Journal of Neurology, Neurosurgery, and Psychiatry* 29: 192–95.

Kidd, K.K. (1984). Stuttering as a genetic disorder. In R.F. Curlee and W.H. Perkins, eds., *The nature and treatment of stuttering: New directions*, pp. 149–169. San Diego: College-Hill Press.

Kimura, D. (1977). Acquisition of a motor skill after left-hemisphere damage. *Brain* 100: 527–42.

———. (1979). Neuromotor mechanisms in the evolution of human communication. In H.D. Steklis and M.J. Raleigh, eds., *Neurobiology of social communication in primates*, pp. 197–219. New York: Academic Press.

———. (1982). Left-hemisphere control of oral and brachial movements and their relation to communication. *Philosophical Transactions of the Royal Society of London* B298: 135–49.

Kimura, D. and Archibald, Y. (1974). Motor functions of the left hemisphere. *Brain* 97: 337–50.

Kinsbourne, M. (1982). Hemisphere specialization and the growth of human understanding. *American Psychologist* 3: 411–20.

Kinsbourne, M. and McMurray, J. (1975). The effect of cerebral dominance on time sharing between speaking and tapping by preschool children. *Child Development* 46: 240–42.

Larsen, B., Skinhoj, E., and Lassen, N.A. (1978). Variations in regional cerebral blood flow in the right and left hemispheres during automatic speech. *Brain* 101: 193–209.

Ley, R.G. and Bryden, M.P. (1982). A dissociation of right and left hemispheric effects for recognizing emotional tone and verbal context. *Brain and Cognition* 1: 3–9.

Liepmann, H. (1908). Die linke Hemisphäre und das Handeln. In *Drei Aufsätze aus dem Apraxiegebiet*, pp. 17–50. Berlin: Springer.

Lomas, J. and Kimura, D. (1976). Intrahemispheric interaction between speaking and sequential manual activity. *Neuropsychologia* 14: 23–33.

Mateer, C.A. (1983). Motor and perceptual functions of the left hemisphere and their interaction. In S. Segalowitz, ed., *Language functions and brain organization*, pp. 145–70. New York: Academic Press.

Mateer, C. and Kimura, D. (1977). Impairment of nonverbal oral movements in aphasia. *Brain and Language* 4: 262–76.

Moore, W.H. (1976). Bilateral tachistoscopic word perception of stutterers and normal subjects. *Brain and Language* 3: 434–42.

———. (1984). Central nervous system characteristics of stutterers. In R.F. Curlee and W.H. Perkins, eds., *The nature and treatment of stuttering: New directions*, pp. 49–66. San Diego: College-Hill Press.

———. (1986). Hemispheric alpha asymmetries of stutterers and nonstutterers for the recall and recognition of words and connected reading passages: Some relationships to severity of stuttering. *Journal of Fluency Disorders* 11: 71–89.

Moore, W.H. and Boberg, E. (1987). Hemispheric processing and stuttering. In L. Rustin, H. Purser and D. Rowley, eds., *Progress in the treatment of fluency disorders*, pp. 19–42. London: Taylor and Francis.

Moore, W.H. and Haynes, W.O. (1980). Alpha hemispheric asymmetry and stuttering: Some support for a segmentation dysfunction hypothesis. *Journal of Speech and Hearing Research* 23: 229–47.

Mountcastle, V.B. (1978). An organizing principle for cerebral function: The unit module and the distributed system. In G.M. Edelman and V.B. Mountcastle, eds., *The mindful brain: Cortical organization and the group-selective theory of higher brain functions*. Cambridge, MA: MIT Press.

Ojemann, G.A. (1983). Brain organization for language from the perspective of electrical stimulation mapping. *The Behavioural and Brain Sciences* 2: 189–230.

Ojemann, G. and Mateer, C.A. (1979). Human language cortex: localization of memory syntax and sequential motor-phoneme identification systems. *Science* 205: 1401–3.

Oke, A., Keller, R., Mefford, I. and Adams, R.N. (1978). Lateralization of norepinephrine in human thalamus. *Science* 200: 1411–13.

Oldfield, R.C. (1971). The assessment and analysis of handedness: The Edinburgh Inventory. *Neuropsychologia* 9: 97–113.

Orton, S.T. (1928). A physiological theory of reading disability and stuttering in children. *New England Journal of Medicine* 199: 1046–52.

Penfield, W. and Welch, K. (1949). The supplementary motor area in the cerebral cortex of man. *Transactions of the American Neurological Association* 74: 79–184.

———. (1951). The supplementary motor area of the cerebral cortex. *Archives of Neurology and Psychiatry* 66: 289–317.

Perkins, W.H. (1985). Horizons and beyond: Confessions of a carpenter. *Seminars in Speech and Language* 6: 233–44.

Peters, M. (1980). Why the preferred hand taps more quickly than the non-preferred hand: Three experiments on handedness. *Canadian Journal of Psychology* 34: 62–71.

———. (1987). A nontrivial motor performance difference between right-handers and left-handers: Attention as intervening variable in the expression of handedness. *Canadian Journal of Psychology* 41: 91–99.

Pool, K., Freeman, F.J. and Finitzo, T. (1987). Brain electrical activity mapping: Applications to vocal motor control disorders. In H.F.M. Peters and W. Hulstijn, eds., *Speech motor dynamics in stuttering*, pp. 151–60. New York: Springer-Verlag.

Preilowski, B. (1975). Bilateral motor interaction: Perceptual-motor performance of partial and complete "split-brain" patients. In K.J. Zulch et al., eds., *Cerebral localization*, pp. 115–32. New York/Heidelberg: Springer-Verlag.

Roland, P.E. (1984). Organization of motor control by the normal human brain. *Human Neurobiology* 2: 205–16.

———. (1985). Cortical organization of voluntary behavior in man. *Human Neurobiology* 4: 155–67.

Roland, P.E., Larsen, B., Lassen, N.A. and Skinhoj, E. (1980). Supplementary motor area and other cortical areas in organization of voluntary movements in man. *Journal of Neurophysiology* 43: 118–36.

Rosenfield, D.B. and Goodglass, H. (1980). Dichotic testing of cerebral dominance of stutterers. *Brain and Language* 11: 170–80.

Ross, E.D. and Mesulam, M.-M. (1979). Dominant language functions of the right hemisphere. *Archives of Neurology* 31: 144–48.

Schaffer, C.E. and Davidson, R.J. (1983). Frontal and parietal electroencephalogram asymmetry in depressed and nondepressed subjects. *Biological Psychiatry* 18: 753–62.

Sheehan, J.G. (1970). *Stuttering: Research and therapy*. New York: Harper and Row.

Sheehan, J.G. and Costley, M.S. (1977). A reexamination of the role of heredity in stuttering. *Journal of Speech and Hearing Disorders* 42: 47–59.

Sperry, R.W. (1974). Lateral specialization in the surgically separated hemispheres. In F.O. Schmitt and F.G. Worden, eds., *The neurosciences: Third study program*, pp. 5–20. Cambridge, MA: MIT Press.

Springer, S.P. (1986). Dichotic listening. In H.J. Hannay, ed., *Experimental techniques in human neuropsychology*, pp. 138–66. New York: Oxford University Press.

Stuss, D.T. and Benson, D.F. (1986). *The frontal lobes*. New York: Raven Press.

Tanji, J., Taniguchi, K. and Saga, T. (1980). Supplementary motor area: Neuronal response to motor instructions. *Journal of Neurophysiology* 43: 60–68.

Todor, J.I. and Kyprie, P.M. (1980). Hand differences in the rate and variability of rapid tapping. *Journal of Motor Behavior* 12: 57–62.

Travis, L.E. (1931). *Speech pathology*. New York: Appleton.

———. (1978). The cerebral dominance theory of stuttering: 1931–1978. *Journal of Speech and Hearing Disorders* 43: 278–81.

Van Riper, C. (1934). A new test of laterality. *Journal of Experimental Psychology* 17: 305–13.

———. (1971). *The nature of stuttering*. Englewood Cliffs, N.J.: Prentice-Hall.

Wada, J.A., Clarke, R., and Hamm, A. (1975). Cerebral hemispheric asymmetry in humans. *Archives of Neurology* 32: 239–46.

Watson, R.T., Shepherd, W., Gonzalez-Rothi, L. and Heilman, K.M. (1986). Apraxia and the supplementary motor area. *Archives of Neurology* 43: 787–92.

Webster, R.L. (1980). Evolution of a target-based behavioral therapy for stuttering. *Journal of Fluency Disorders* 5: 303–20.

Webster, W.G. (1985). Neuropsychological models of stuttering—I. Representation of sequential response mechanisms. *Neuropsychologia* 23: 263–67.

———. (1986a). Response sequence organization and reproduction by stutterers. *Neuropsychologia* 24: 813–21.

———. (1986b). Neuropsychological models of stuttering—II. Interhemispheric interference. *Neuropsychologia* 24: 737–41.

———. (1987). Rapid letter transcription performance by stutterers. *Neuropsychologia* 25: 845–47.

———. (1988). Neural mechanisms underlying stuttering: Evidence from bimanual handwriting. *Brain and Language* 33: 226–44.

———. (1989a). Sequence initiation by stutterers under conditions of response competition. *Brain and Language* 36: 286–300.

———. (1989b). Sequence reproduction deficits in stutterers tested under non-speeded response conditions. *Journal of Fluency Disorders* 14: 79–86.

————. (1990a). Concurrent cognitive processing and letter transcription deficits in stutterers. *Canadian Journal of Psychology* 44: 1–13

————. (1990b). Evidence in bimanual finger tapping of an attentional component to stuttering. *Behavioural Brain Research* 37: 93–100

Webster, W.G. and Poulos, M. (1987). Handedness distributions among adults who stutter. *Cortex* 23: 705–8.

————. (1989). *Facilitating Fluency: Transfer strategies for adult stuttering treatment programs.* Tucson, Arizona: Communication Skill Builders, Inc.

Wiesendanger, M. (1986). Initiation of voluntary movements and the supplementary motor area. In H. Heuer and C. Fromm, eds., *Generation and modulation of action patterns, Experimental Brain Research,* Vol. 15, pp. 3–13. New York: Springer-Verlag.

Wingate, M.E. (1964). A standard definition of stuttering. *Journal of Speech and Hearing Disorders* 29: 484–89.

Wise, S.P. (1984). The nonprimary motor cortex and its role in the cerebral control of movement. In G.M. Edelman, W.E. Gall and W.M. Cowan, eds., *Dynamic aspects of neocortical function,* pp. 525–55. New York: John Wiley and Sons.

Wolff, P.H., Hurwitz, I. and Moss, H. (1977). Serial organization of motor skills in left- and right-handed adults. *Neuropsychologia* 15: 539–46.

Wood, F., Stump, D., McKennhan, A., Sheldon, S. and Proctor, J. (1980). Patterns of regional cerebral blood flow during attempted reading aloud by stutterers both on and off haloperidol medication: Evidence for inadequate left frontal activation during stuttering. *Brain and Language* 9: 141–44.

Zimmerman, G. (1980). Stuttering: A disorder of movement. *Journal of Speech and Hearing Research* 23: 122–36.

Discussion

A. Caruso: I want to start off by saying that there was a very enthusiastic response to your presentation. It was very well received. Our group felt that you presented a number of complicated issues in a very clear manner and they appreciated the way in which it was presented. An additional comment was that one of the hallmarks of your work, which cannot be said of a lot of research, is that in your models and theories you make a real attempt to incorporate both the psyche and the soma of stuttering. That may be more difficult to do but we believe it is reality.

One of the questions from our group was whether there was any overlap in the performance on your tasks, between the stutterers and nonstutterers? If there was, could you comment on that? If there were normal subjects who performed similarly to some stutterers, what was their speech like?

W. Webster: Certainly there was overlap. One of the characteristics of these kinds of performance measures is that there are some subjects with extreme scores in both directions. There were some stutterers who were really very poor. I alluded to this briefly in my discussion of repetitive sequential finger tapping in which I found 2 of 18 stutterers, and subsequently others, who simply could not do the task. We would demonstrate the sequence, and by the time we started the trial several seconds later, they could not remember what they were to do. The other

stutterers, on the other hand, were really very good at the tapping. In fact, overall on this particular task, the groups were
very similar. The group differences were evident in the
sequence reproduction task and the various bimanual tasks.
Again, there was variation within each group, and there was
overlap between the groups in the distributions.

I cannot tell you anything about the speech of either the stutterers or the control subjects because I did not do speech assessments. In this initial work I decided to treat stuttering as a categorical self-defined variable and to focus on aspects of manual
motor performance that I thought would tell me something
about brain organization in people who stutter. This was also
convenient in that I am not a speech-language pathologist. I
think that the research has now reached the stage where it is
imperative that I begin to relate speech performance to those
measures of manual motor performance which are supposedly
indicative of one or another aspect of brain function. I would
certainly hope to develop some collaboration with a speech-
language pathologist to do that in the future.

In terms of a variation among stutterers, I cannot tell you as
much as I might like to. The issue of subgroups is certainly of
interest to me and I have alluded to it in some of my published
work. Given that I think these motor performance tasks tell us
something about brain mechanisms, it follows that I expect that
ultimately these kinds of tasks will be of utility in differentiating
subgroups of stutterers with respect to etiology. One working
hypothesis I want to explore relates to family history, and this is
an outgrowth of a study that my colleague, Marie Poulos, has
been doing. She went back over nearly 170 consecutive clients
who have come through the Rehabilitation Centre in Ottawa for
stuttering assessment and treatment. Two-thirds reported a
family history of stuttering. What was especially interesting
about her data was that among those without a family history of
stuttering, nearly 40% reported some physical trauma that had
occurred in early childhood and that could potentially have pre-
cipitated stuttering. These incidents included head injuries, gen-

eral anesthetics, and birth complications. Virtually none (2%) of the stutterers with a family history reported any such incident. The data were remarkably similar to those published more than 50 years ago by West, Nelson and Berry (1939). Bohme's (1968) data make it clear that stuttering can result from early brain damage but is not an inevitable consequence of it. Of his 313 cases with normal intelligence, 24% stuttered. Whether or not a particular occurrence of early brain damage results in stuttering presumably depends on which particular neural systems have been compromised, how they have been compromised, and the extent of the compromise. Presumably within the subgroup of stutterers with no family history of stuttering but reporting early trauma, there will be considerable variation in the underlying neurological mechanisms. Presumably these mechanisms may differ from those underlying stuttering in those with a family history and genetic predisposition. And I would certainly expect this variation to be reflected in motor performance tasks that are supposedly indicative of inter- and intra-hemispheric processes.

A Caruso: When you use the term attention, are you implying a high level of consciousness, controlled attention, or is it more automatic?

W. Webster: I am using the term to imply a more automatic process, although that does not mean it cannot be compensated for or brought under some voluntary control. I am using the term to be generally synonymous with hemispheric activation. What I am suggesting is that instead of there being a sustained activation of the left hemisphere or an inherent bias towards left hemisphere activation, as many have argued one finds in normal right-handers, activation in stutterers is labile and shifts readily, possibly like that of left-handers. What underlies these shifts is an important issue, but I do not conceptualize it as being a matter of conscious control.

A. Caruso: How do you think anxiety would affect performance on these tasks?

W. Webster: That is an interesting question and one I would like to explore. To the extent that anxiety involves greater right hemisphere activation, one would expect more interhemispheric overflow and hence right hand (left hemisphere) performance should deteriorate on bimanual tasks. I think that is a clear prediction, and it would be informative to test it out.

A. Caruso: As we have talked about it a little bit, I would like to inject one comment here. Anxiety, as it has been looked at, in non-speech literature, is apparently a "U" shaped function. There is a level or degree of anxiety that causes performance to break down, if you will, and there is another level or degree of anxiety that seems to enhance performance. Is there room in your model to suggest that some degree of anxiety would actually increase performance in some of these incidents?

W. Webster: If one equates anxiety with arousal or hemispheric activation, then increased levels of anxiety may be associated with differentially increased levels of right and left hemisphere activation. With very low levels of arousal, there would not be right hemisphere interference with the left, but the left hemisphere system might be inadequately primed. With moderate levels of anxiety, the increased left hemisphere activation might in some sense focus attention on the motoric aspects of the task with the right hemisphere not sufficiently activated to overflow. With higher levels of arousal, left hemisphere sequencing may be interfered with both by interhemispheric as well as intra-hemispheric processes. In summary, yes, I could imagine that some degree of anxiety might increase rather than decrease performance, but I see no reason to expect those increases to favour the stutterer differentially over the nonstutterer. There are other situations in which I could better imagine such differential facilitation; specifically, certain tasks that require rapid shifts of attention between the hemispheres.

A. Caruso: My group would like you to review how you arrived at the conclusion and implication of the supplementary motor area? Could you state your rationale in the logical thinking process that you went through when you implicated that?

W. Webster: It draws upon analogical reasoning and the parallels between the behavioral effects we have been observing in stutterers and the kinds of functions thought to be mediated by supplementary motor area (SMA). The line of argument started with the evidence of an overlap between speech and nonspeech motor processes. I think this is most clearly seen in cerebral blood flow studies which demonstrate SMA involvement in the planning and organization of speech and nonspeech movements, but not the actual execution of the movement. Given the manual sequencing impairments we have found, the overlap of speech and nonspeech processing makes SMA a candidate for being an area involved in stuttering. Secondly, the place where stutterers have their problems in finger tapping is with the planning, organization, and initiation of new response sequences, not the execution of well practiced ones. Again that sounds very similar to the inferences about SMA that have been made on the basis of cerebral blood flow studies. The other thing that caught my attention initially was the results of the bimanual handwriting study in which we found in stutterers more frequently reversed letters written by the left hand. Not only does the SMA have very extensive interhemispheric connections, but damage to it in nonhuman primates results in mirror image movements by the two limbs. In other words when the integrity of the SMA has been compromised, independent limb and hand movements are reduced, as in stutterers. It is an effect that is ameliorated by sectioning of the callosum.

I think these were the three major reasons I started to look seriously at the SMA, and which in turn led me to think about a more general frontal lobe involvement involving attentional processes.

A. Caruso: We noticed that you really zeroed in on the SMA, rather than implicating the connections between SMA and some other major areas, perhaps the basal ganglia, perhaps others and that was really the thought behind the question. One final comment from our group. We found your clinical implications to be somewhat, if not more than somewhat, depressing.

W. Webster: In what way?

A. Caruso: The fact that there are no changes, no cures. The fact that fluency will only maintain itself with the active use of controls. There are some people who have done longstanding, direct, clinical work and who can identify cases where this would not be true, even with adult stutterers. I am wondering if you could comment on that, if you could lift some of my depression?

W. Webster: I think that whether your depression is justified depends ultimately on what may underlie the fragility and what one is looking for with treatment. If there is a lesion or mis-wiring of the system, and if you are looking for a cure, then perhaps some pessimism is warranted. If there is a neurotransmitter problem, then perhaps less so as there are factors that increasingly are coming to be recognized as being able to affect the synthesis or breakdown of neurotransmitters. This is why I began to think about my experiences with sugar and how sugar might be having its effects on my speech. If you are prepared to accept the idea of control rather than cure, then I think there is a basis for optimism. I suggested earlier that stuttering severity is influenced by right hemisphere activation. I think it is increasingly clear that there are behavioural techniques that can provide a vehicle for bringing that right hemisphere more under control, hence reducing some of the extreme ups and downs. But there will continue to be an unstable speech motor control system that can deteriorate.

A. Caruso: But you do not feel that changes in the speech behaviour itself can bring about changes in the neuroprocesses underlying that behaviour or that those changed neuroprocesses become, for lack of a better term, stabilized?

W. Webster: Absolutely. It is not just behaviour that emerges from brain function, but brain function that emerges from behaviour. Success in speech leads to improved confidence and reduced apprehension, and I am sure that a less volatile right hemisphere goes hand in hand with that. I am also sure that as speech techniques such as rate control and gentle onsets are practiced and become more automatic, the left hemisphere speech motor control systems are themselves stabilized. In other words, I have no difficulty with the idea that as a person systematically attacks avoidances, practices speech in new and varied situations, and achieves successes in controlling fluency, stuttering severity diminishes and it becomes easier to maintain control, and that the reasons for this can be understood in neuropsychological terms. And this happens because of changes in the physiology of the system. But at the same time, I think the system remains inherently unstable or fragile and can deteriorate very readily.

R. Kroll: On behalf of our blue group I would also like to thank you for a most informative, if somewhat provocative, kind of presentation. Most stimulating, well organized, with a lot of information. I would like to begin by, perhaps, continuing on a question that Tony was asking. If stuttering cannot be reversed, as you mentioned, how do you explain or how do you account for the so-called permanent recovery, the high-rate of permanent recovery in young children? Does this imply, and would you be willing to suggest, that there is some degree of plasticity in the brain at an early age beyond which this does not occur?

W. Webster: There are two or three points I would make in response to this. First, I would stress that my research so far has dealt only with adults. It may well be that my research participants were the children who would not have been successful in treatment. Maybe adults who stutter were as children at the upper end of a distribution of system fragility or instability, and those children who showed spontaneous recovery were at the lower end, or perhaps were qualitatively different in terms of underlying mechanisms. There may well be more than one type of stuttering not only in adults, as I suggested earlier, but even more types of stuttering in children. Perhaps only those children who have the kinds of neurological anomalies I have been suggesting will continue to stutter into adulthood. This again brings me back to my interest in the issue of subgroups.

But suppose, hypothetically, the basic problem of the system relates to a process like myelinization. Suppose that for many children there is insufficient differentiation among the columns due to a lack of myelinization. The myelinization process continues, but it is delayed. It might continue to be a problem only in those individuals for whom the myelinization process was never quite complete. It might also be that even for some of the children in whom the myelinization process is not completed and who do not have normal degree of functional differentiation among columns, there may be behavioral or cognitive processes that accomplish the same thing. That gets me back to the earlier comments about cognitive organization. Perhaps through exposing children to certain experiences they learn how to organize their speech planning processes so that it has the result of increasing functional differentiation.

R. Kroll: Much of what you are saying, in terms of the sequential finger-tapping studies and other studies that you have done, indicates that stutterers have difficulty doing two motor tasks, two separate motor tasks, simultaneously. In therapy we often ask stutterers to monitor two specific motor behaviours, such as gentle onsets and prolonged speech, simultaneously or alternatively. One of the complaints that clinicians often get from stutterers is that it is difficult for them to think about what they are going to say and how they are going to say it. How would you explain our current clinical methodology in light of your model? Can we really justify it?

W. Webster: Your experience is very similar to that of Marie Poulos with whom I work, and I agree this is a problem. One of the things you might want to do is to try to make some of the components of social interaction more automatic than they are to begin with. For example, if you have someone who has avoided personal introductions, it will be very difficult for him to monitor speech while attempting at the same time to generate a social script for introductions. But if he can first rehearse what the social scripts are for introductions so they become somewhat practiced and automatic, then more attention or cognitive capacity can be directed at speech monitoring during the social interaction itself. But as soon as the social demands become unpredictable or less automatic, then monitoring ability may fall down. This is also the reason for trying to have clients practice their skills all the time so the skills become increasingly automatic. Then when socially difficult situations arise, they can deal with them while still maintaining fluency skills.

R. Kroll: I would like to provide you with a hypothetical case scenario. You are presented with a chronic avoider, someone who has an almost phobic reaction to certain speech situations, who is, to use an older term, an interiorized stutterer. If we adopt your model we would engage primarily in nonavoidance therapy to smooth out the right hemisphere activation. Yet many of us in our group, myself included, have had very successful experience with fluency shaping strategies with these people. Are you comfortable with that?

W. Webster: Yes, I think fluency shaping should work well in such a case. One of the reasons the person is interiorized, skirting around and avoiding words and sentences, is that he can anticipate the problems he is going to have. It would seem to me that desensitization and fluency shaping would go hand in hand. The fluency shaping helps the person use the left hemisphere to its full capability and there is no longer a need to avoid those words. Desensitization contributes in that it lowers right hemisphere activation, reducing potential interference with the left hemisphere mechanisms.

R. Kroll: Several of us, including Dr. Yeudall, were concerned with the link that you have been making. Dr. Yeudall pointed out that the hands are not homotopically connected to the callosal system. How do you feel this impacts on your assertion and the conclusions you are drawing?

W. Webster: Dr. Yeudall is quite correct. But as I said earlier in the presentation, the interhemispheric connections between the hands all go through the supplementary motor area. They do not go directly from the primary motor area of one hemisphere to the primary motor area of the other. It is because of the lack of homotopic connections in the primary motor areas that we need to be thinking about the supplementary motor area.

R. Kroll: Just one final quick question, a point of clarification. Was it the nondominant hand that showed the interference effects in stutterers in your concurrent finger-tapping experiments?

W. Webster: In the concurrent task experiments, I focused on the dominant right hand doing the repetitive sequential finger tapping and the sequence reproduction task and the nondominant left hand doing the concurrent task. In the bimanual handwriting task the focus was on the two hands together. In that particular task we tried to make it language oriented led by the left hemisphere. We did this by presenting four words on every trial and the task was to write the first letter of the words. Our main focus of attention was then on overflow from the preferred hand (which we thought would write in the correct orientation) to the nonpreferred hand.

H. Gregory: One of the things we would like you to address some more are the implications for therapy of the findings from your research and your theorizing. You also heard Dr. Moore this morning. I know that if I were you, I would be thinking what kind of implications he is drawing and how might those be like mine or different from mine? Some of the group heard Dr. Moore imply that increases in transition time in speech increase right hemisphere processes. Were you saying something different?

W. Webster: Yes, I think you are right. This is one area where Dr. Moore and I may part company. My inclination, which probably reflects a background in comparative neuropsychology rather than linguistics, has been to see how far I can go in understanding the system and processes without invoking linguistic concepts. Right now I am not persuaded that such concepts have to be introduced. But I nonetheless think that the question of what different skills entail in terms of hemispheric activation is a most interesting one, and one that may ultimately contribute to our understanding of how different factors affect stuttering.

H. Gregory: Research has been done comparing nonspeech reaction time and coordination of the speech mechanism and speech reaction time and coordination of the speech mechanism. Dr. Luper has done some of this research. We wondered about extrapolating from nonspeech coordination activity to your hypothesis about the speech mechanism and stuttering?

W. Webster: The literature on speech reaction times is quite clear; people who stutter have slower onset times. In the case of nonspeech reaction times, in tasks like finger reaction times, the literature is very contradictory. There are some studies that report problems, and some do not. A graduate student, Lynn Ryan, and I undertook a study of manual reaction times in an attempt to resolve some of the discrepancies. The work was a partial test of a general hypothesis that group differences in reaction times reflect task complexity. In the initial study we varied decision complexity but kept response complexity more or less constant by comparing groups of stutterers and nonstutterers on simple, two-choice, and four-choice reaction time procedures. We also varied decision complexity with a four-choice reaction time procedure with and without spatial contiguity between stimulus and response locus. In neither comparison did we find the expected Group x Complexity interaction. Instead the stutterers were slower than nonstutterers in initiating and completing responses on all task conditions. I now want to do the converse study of keeping decision complexity constant but varying response complexity, and frankly I expect to find a Group x Complexity interaction under those conditions. However, I am not so sure that that will help resolve the discrepancies in the literature on this matter.

But to go back to the question, I do not have an answer at this time for the discrepancies in the literature on manual reaction times except to attribute them to implicit or explicit task demands, but that is not terribly satisfying.

H. Gregory: Would it be appropriate in this kind of research to also have measures on some coordinative aspects of the stutterers' speech.

W. Webster: Absolutely. As I was saying in response to an earlier question, I think that I must now include some speech measures. I think I have gone as far as I should just looking at nonspeech processes.

H. Gregory: One last intriguing question. What recommendations would you have to improve finger-tapping? Are there relationships between what you would recommend to improve finger tapping and what you would do for the stutterers?

W. Webster: Maybe that goes back to my answer to Dr. Kroll's ques-
· tion about the need to try to make as much of this process as automatic as possible, through practice in as many situations as possible. Whether it ever becomes fully automatic is a very big question.

Questions from the Floor

L. Lavallee: I have a question regarding the origin of stuttering. With reference to a genetic base, you support this by the fact that it runs in families. Others have stated that there is an emotional cause to stuttering, that there might be a high parental concern for stuttering. Given that you have said that stuttering can be reversed by therapy in a positive way, might the brain be plastic enough to be affected in a negative way by some of the variables I have already mentioned?

W. Webster: I see no reason in principle that that could not be the case. Brain development reflects both genetic factors as well as environmental ones. I could certainly imagine how sustained right hemisphere overactivation brought about through negative emotion, combined with uncertainty and conflict, could have a permanently destabilizing effect on what would have otherwise been a normal fluent system. We see dysfluencies in nonstutterers under conditions of extreme stress or uncertainty, and perhaps if such dysfluencies occur sufficiently often in the child with a developing brain, there will be a permanent alteration in the sensitivity of the system to future disruptions.

B. Johnston: I was wondering if you could comment on the research that Sandra Witelson has been doing on the corpus callosum. I believe her research has shown that it is larger in left-handers and in women. Would that have any implications in this model?

W. Webster: I could indeed imagine implications, and that is why I included both left-handers and females in the study on bimanual handwriting. Unfortunately I found nothing in my data to differentiate male and female stutterers, or even right- and left-handers with respect to the pattern of overflow effects. I should comment that there is some controversy about the reliability and the significance of sex and handedness differences in callosal size, and so the implications of the lack of sex and hand effects in my study are unclear.

In trying to understand sex differences in stuttering, I am more inclined to focus on intrahemispheric neuronal organization rather than interhemispheric processes. As Dr. Mateer discussed last evening, there is evidence that females have a more focal type of neuronal organization in the left hemisphere than do males. In males, the speech and language systems seem to be more diffusely organized, as evidenced by the fact that damage almost anywhere in the left hemisphere has a reasonable probability of resulting in aphasia and apraxia. In females, on the other hand, the damage has to include the anterior region for there to be aphasic and apraxic effects. It seems to be that if you think about the idea of peri-columnar inhibition, perhaps the more focally organized the columns, the closer they are together, the less the opportunity for interference. If the columns are distributed, then intuitively it would seem that there would be more opportunity for interference from activity in other interspersed columns. Maybe in males the columns do not inhibit one another as much as in females because they are more distant, and that may underlie the apparently greater vulnerability of males to stuttering. I do not know what the answer is, but again I find it easier to think of sex differences in stuttering in these terms rather than in those of callosal fibres, particularly in light of the contradictory morphology literature.

C. Mateer: I want to ask two questions, if I may, and also want to compliment you on a fine talk. One of my questions concerns your reference to the work of Doreen Kimura, with regard to

her theoretic formulations of left hemisphere control for movement. Part of that theory is that the left hemisphere controls not
just contralateral hand movement, but ipsilateral hand movement, to a certain extent, as well. After left hemisphere lesions,
individuals may show an apraxia with their left hand. Since a
lot of the disruption you were describing has to do with distur-
bances in the left hand, how much of that could be simply
another manifestation of this left hemisphere incapability, in
stutterers, for control? It was not quite clear in all the studies
whether everything had been counterbalanced and everything
had been done with both hands. I was thinking of the tasks that
involved the bimanual activities or single manual activities
with the left hand.

W. Webster: In terms of unimanual performance on the sequence
reproduction task, we tested both the right and left hands individually and stutterers were impaired with both hands. We
interpreted those findings as reflecting impaired left hemisphere motor sequence organization in stutterers. In terms of
the concurrent bimanual performance, and perhaps I could
focus on the repetitive sequential finger tapping combined with
knob turning or button pressing, stutterers were not impaired
on the component tasks, only when the tasks were performed
together. In that study we completely counterbalanced conditions and included both right hand finger tapping with left
hand knob turning and left hand finger tapping with right
hand knob turning. It was only in the former condition that we
found differential losses between stutterers and nonstutterers.
It seemed to me that indicated that the stutterers were not generally more impaired when doing any two concurrent tasks,
but it was related to the particular pattern of hands and task
demands. Of course the left hand finger sequential tapping
combined with right hand knob turning is neuropsychologically ambiguous.

   I do not think I am really addressing your question satisfac-
torily because it has been a while since I thought that issue

through. Perhaps in light of the hour I could beg off that question, but I will think about it and get back to you individually.

C. Mateer: I tried to think about it too and could not come up with any answers. I just wondered if you had thought about it. I like the idea of looking at a very molecular level, a very minute level, at possible discontrol mechanisms. Certainly what we have learned about visual systems or auditory systems is greatly enhanced by looking at the cellular or neuronal level and looking at this common organization. It strikes me that in seizure disorders, which is really modeled as a lack of inhibition among those columns, what causes the seizuring activity is an unbridled lack of inhibition across neurons in different columns. It seems to me, just from a motor point of view, that we are seeing the same kind of phenomenon. Have you thought about that?

W. Webster: No, I have not thought about that at all. Your comments are very interesting, and I would like to consider them.

C. Mateer: Some of the antiseizure medications, presumably boost the inhibitory effect among the adjacent neurons.

W. Webster: Everyone asks me if ultimately there will be some medication that cures stuttering. Perhaps one of these anti-seizure medications will be it but frankly I would not count on speech therapists being put out of business quite yet.

References
Bohme, G. (1968). Stammering and cerebral lesions in early childhood. Examination of 802 children and adults with cerebral lesions. *Folia Phoniatrica* 20: 239–49.

West, R., Nelson, S. and Berry, M. (1939). The heredity of stuttering. *Quarterly Journal of Speech* 25: 23–30.

Lorne T. Yeudall, Laura Manz, Cathy Ridenour
Akio Tani, John Lind, Orestes Fedora

4 Variability in the Central Nervous System of Stutterers

Introduction

In 1984 a neuropsychological theory, based on a three-dimensional functional model of the brain, was presented at the Banff conference on stuttering behavior (Yeudall, 1985). The major tenets of the theory focus on the hierarchical and dynamic nature of brain organization and postulate that different brain systems are involved in speech production. It was proposed that compromised functioning of one or more of these brain systems, in part, is responsible for stuttering behavior and its heterogeneity. The theory accounts for some of the attributes of stutterers (e.g., sex differences, age of onset, effects of stress, normal singing, etc.). The theory is multidimensional in nature and attempts to integrate physiological (e.g., phylogenetic, ontogenetic, neurological, neurohormonal, neurochemical and neurotransmitter systems) and experiential factors within a developmental framework for a given individual. The multidimensionality of the theory, in terms of brain function, addresses some of the inadequacies in previous research pointed out by Rosenfield and Nudelman (1987), such as looking for the "single" cause for stuttering, accounting for the mechanism or the effects of stress or anxiety, or considering stuttering as some "supra-brain" event.

Boberg and Yeudall (1985), in a preliminary study, compared two persistent and two controlled stutterers to a large age matched control group (N=58) on variables from a comprehensive assessment battery consisting of neuropsychological, brainstem evoked potential and quantitative EEG variables. The controlled stutterers essentially had normal neuropsychological performance, whereas the persistent stutterers had a significant number of impaired scores. Quantitative analysis of EEG (qEEG) during the performance of a spatial task revealed excessive alpha power in the posterior regions of both hemispheres and in the frontal regions of the right hemisphere. Of particular interest, three of the four stutterers, including both controlled stutterers, showed significantly shortened interpeak latencies for the right brainstem auditory evoked response. This latter finding is consistent with views of compromised functioning of the brainstem in stutterers (Hall and Jerger, 1978; Rosenfield and Jerger, 1984; and Zimmerman, 1984).

Manz (1988) selected a set of neuropsychological variables, primarily sensitive to the functional integrity of the frontal lobes, to predict treatment outcome in 17 stutterers. Four neuropsychological variables were predictive of post-treatment frequency of stuttering, two of post-treatment rate of speech and two of post-treatment attitude towards speech. These very preliminary findings suggested a possible relationship between the degree of neuropsychological impairment and the severity of stuttering. Examination of her individual subjects, compared to a control data base, revealed that the majority showed significant impairments for one or more of the neuropsychological measures sensitive to the motor systems of the frontal lobes. Variability was evident among her stutterers' neuropsychological performances with three showing a different pattern of impaired scores, when compared to the other stutterers.

The present study examines the variability in stutterers pertaining to severity and levels of involvement of different brain systems (e.g., brainstem, midbrain, thalamus/basal ganglia, cerebellar and cortical). From a theoretical perspective, stuttering behavior is viewed as the dynamic interaction of these different brain systems involving the cortical motor systems of the frontal lobes and associated subcortical structures, including the limbic system (Crosson and Hughs, 1987; Yeudall, 1985).

Method

Assessment Strategy

The functional integrity of the cortical regions of the two cerebral hemispheres was assessed by neuropsychological variables which focus on evaluating the frontal regions of the brain (Yeudall et al., 1986). Galambos 40 Hz and other middle latency responses were used in the assessment of midbrain/thalamic/cortical functions (Galambos et al., 1981; Kraus et al., 1982; Kraus et al., 1988; Picton et al., 1974; Spydell et al., 1985; Woods et al., 1987). The functional integrity of the brainstem was assessed through the use of standard clinical auditory brainstem evoked potentials (i.e., interpeak latency differences) as well as a stressor condition involving increased auditory stimulation rates (Lasky, 1984). Quantitative analysis of the EEG (qEEG) was conducted to obtain a dynamic measure of brain function reflecting hemispheric activity during actual speech production (Pockberger et al., 1985).

Subjects

The majority of subjects (13/17) were clients who attended an intensive three-week clinic at the Institute for Stuttering Treatment and Research (ISTAR) in Edmonton, Alberta. Three of the remaining subjects were private clients of the senior author while the fourth subject attended an intensive clinic elsewhere. The mean age of the 17 stutterers was 33.5 years with a range from 17 to 55 years. The sample consisted of 12 males and 5 females; a ratio of 2.4 to 1, respectively. The average Full Scale IQ of the stutterers was 108.4 with no significant difference between the Verbal (106.36) and Performance (110.86) Scales. Handedness as measured by the Annett's Handedness Questionnaire (Annett, 1970) revealed that all 17 stutterers were right handed.

Assessment Procedures

Neuropsychological, intellectual, and qEEG assessments were performed at ISTAR and the Department of Neuropsychology, Alberta

Hospital, Edmonton. Brainstem auditory evoked potential assessments were conducted at the Department of Audiology, University of Alberta Hospital, Edmonton for 7 of the stutterers and the remaining 10 were conducted at the Department of Neuropsychology at Alberta Hospital Edmonton. In addition to brainstem evoked potentials, 10 stutterers were assessed using two middle latency procedures at Alberta Hospital, whereas the other 7 stutterers were administered a stress condition as part of the brainstem assessment at the University of Alberta Hospital.

Brainstem Auditory Evoked Potentials (BAEPs)

All auditory evoked potential measures performed at Alberta Hospital, Edmonton, were recorded while the subject was in a reclining position in a comfortable dental chair inside a double wall Industrial Acoustic Chamber (IAC). A Nicolet CA1000 was used to collect auditory brainstem responses which were evoked by rarefaction clicks of 0.1 msec duration presented at 75 to 85 dB nHL at a rate of 11.8 per second. Simultaneous ipsilateral and contralateral recordings, using C_z as the active lead and ipsilateral and contralateral mastoids as the reference leads, were collected using bandpass filters set at 200–3000 Hz with a time base of 10 msec, and a resolution of 0.04 msec. Each response, based on 1500–2000 sweeps, was replicated. The averaged data was transferred to a Data General MV 7800 mini-computer for storage and analysis. Interpeak I-III, III-V and I-V latencies were derived from the absolute latencies for right and left brainstem recordings. The interpeak values and right minus left interpeak differences for each stutterer were compared to a normal control data base (n=100) for which the 99% confidence limits (p=<.05) had been calculated (Fedora, Yeudall and Lind, 1987). Two additional scores reflecting brainstem functioning were derived from the stressor condition; the absolute value of wave V during a stimulation rate of 89.1 per sec, and the latency difference of wave V between the two stimulation rates (10.1 vs 89.1). Both scores were compared to control scores, with lower and upper latency cutoffs.

Middle Latency Procedures

Galambos 40 Hz. The 40 Hz evoked response was elicited by rarefaction clicks presented independently to the left and right ears at a rate of 40/sec at 75 dB for 1000 sweeps. The time base was 100 msec with the bandpass filters set at 5–100 Hz. The responses were recorded over the left posterior inferior frontal region (F_7), overlapping Broca's region, and its homologous region of the right hemisphere (F_8), the mid-temporal regions (T_3 and T_4), superior central motor regions (C_3 and C_4) and the superior parietal regions (P_3 and P_4) referenced to the ipsilateral mastoid (two responses; A_1 with F_7, T_3, C_3, and P_3, and A_2 with F_8, T_4, C_4, and P_4). The criteria for abnormal Galambos 40 Hz responses in order of importance were: 1) a phase shift of the response, 2) the disintegration of the response, 3) a significant attenuation of the amplitude of the response, and 4) abnormalities present for both left and right ear stimulation.

Middle Latency Response. The second procedure used to assess possible subcortical dysfunction was the Middle Latency Response (MLR). This response was evoked by rarefaction clicks presented at a rate of 9.3 per sec for 1000 sweeps with a time base of 90 msecs. The bandpass filters were set at 5–250 Hz. The evoked waveforms (latency and amplitude of Pa) were recorded over the left central region (C_3), right central region (C_4), and C_z. The criteria for abnormal MLR significant asymmetry in amplitude and delayed Pa and Pb latencies.

Neuropsychological Variables

The neuropsychological measures were selected on the basis of their hypothesized sensitivity to the cortical systems of the frontal lobes (Royce, Yeudall and Bock, 1976). They were categorized as being more sensitive to either the left or right hemisphere (even though performance is influenced bilaterally) and to interhemispheric influences. The variables in each category are sequentially ordered as to their considered sensitivity from the anterior to the posterior regions of the frontal lobes (see Table 4.1). A clinical neuropsychological diagnosis implicating compromised functioning of the frontal lobes was made for each stutterer. The diagnosis was based on the individual showing a significant number of deficits covarying in a meaningful pattern consistent with brain-behavior relationships. The results of the clinical assessment of each stutterer is presented by cluster membership. Fourteen of the 17 stutterers were administered the Wechsler Adult Intelligence Scale–Revised (WAIS–R). The Neuropsychological Test Battery was administered in a standardized order by certified psychometricians.

Quantitative Analysis of the EEG (qEEG)

The final assessment of central nervous system function consisted of quantitative analysis of the electroencephalogram (qEEG) which was recorded in another double wall IAC acoustic chamber while the subject relaxed in an Easy-boy chair. The EEG data was collected during expressive speech production and the performance of a spatial task. Speech was elicited using the Oral Word Fluency Test, which requires subjects to generate a maximum number of words in one minute, for the letters F, A and S. The performance of a spatial task consisted of Block Design from the WAIS-R. Eight channels of artifact free EEG were collected using the international 10–20 system (Fp_1-F_z, Fp_2-F_z, T_3-F_z, T_4-F_z, F_7-C_z, F_8-C_z, P_3-C_z, and P_4-C_z) while the subject performed these two tasks. A Texas Instrument 980B computer was used for data acquisition and storage on a 9-track tape (see Boberg and Yeudall, 1985, for more details). The EEG data was then transferred to a Data General MV7800 for further visual editing of artifacts (EMG, eye movement, eye blinks) and 30 one sec epochs for each of the two tasks constituted the data used for quantitative analysis of the EEG.

The measure selected for analysis of the EEG was the degree of coherency between pairs of electrodes within a hemisphere and between hemispheres. Coherence between two electrodes (i.e., brain regions) is interpreted in the same way as the well known product moment correlation. Coherence assumes a value between zero and one with values close to one indicating a strong linear relationship

Table 4.1   Neuropsychology Variables

Left Hemisphere

Wisconsin Card Sorting Test: Errors	(WCST:E)
Wisconsin Card Sorting Test: Subtests	(WCST:S)
Tactual Performance Test: Right	(TPT:R)
Trail Making B	(TMB)
Symbol Digit: Oral	(SD:0)
Symbol Digit: Written	(SD:W)
Purdue Pegboard: Right	(PP:R)
Oral Word Fluency	(OWF)
Written Word Fluency	(WWF)
Name Writing: Right	(NW:R)
Finger Tapping: Right	(FT:R)
Dynamometer: Right	(D:R)

Right Hemisphere

Halstead Category Test	(HCT)
Tactual Performance Test: Left	(TPT:L)
Symbol Gestalt	(SG)
Trail Making A	(TMA)
Purdue Pegboard: Left	(PP:L)
Name Writing: Left	(NW:L)
Finger Tapping: Left	(FT:L)
Dynamometer: Left	(D:L)

Interhemisheric

Tactual Performance Test: Both	(TPT:B)
Purdue Pegboard: Assemblies	(PP:A)
Purdue Pegboard: Both	(PP:B)

between the two electrodes, and values near zero indicating little or no relationship between the electrodes. The degree of coherency between two electrodes or brain regions is considered to reflect the extent of neural communication between them (Gotman, 1987; Lieb et al., 1987). Coherency is usually evaluated across a range of frequencies, with one coherence value calculated for each frequency, providing what is often called the coherence spectrum (Brillinger, 1981). Because of the small number of subjects a reduced number of variables were selected for analysis and consisted of the ratio of homologous electrode pairs between the two hemispheres. For example, the coherency between Fp_1 and F_7 of the left frontal cortex provides an index of the correlated activity between two specific regions of the brain which overlaps Broca's area. Coherency between these two regions (Fp_1 and F_7) of the left hemisphere were then contrasted to coherency pairings from the homologous region of right hemisphere (Fp_2 and F_8) during speech production. Consequently, a ratio of left/right coherencies would provide a measure of hemispheric communication for different regions of the two hemispheres during different cognitive conditions.

Fluency Assessment

Stuttering frequency and speaking rate were measured in two videotaped conditions, reading and conversing with a stranger, before and after a three-week intensive therapy program (Boberg and Kully, 1985). Stuttering frequency was measured by counting the total number of fluent and stuttered syllables spoken and then calculating the percentage of syllables stuttered in each condition and averaging the results. Speaking rate was measured by calculating the number of syllables spoken per minute in each condition and averaging the results.

Data Analysis

Cluster Analysis of Neuropsychological Variables

Cluster analysis of the neuropsychological variables was selected to identify possible subgroups among stutterers, as previous work had demonstrated substantial variability among stutterers for these variables (Boberg and Yeudall, 1985 and Manz, 1988). The cluster analysis was performed using Ward's Method (Ward, 1963), and the SPSS/PC+ program library. A five-cluster solution appeared to be the best solution based on the examination of similarities among individuals within any given cluster. Cluster I consisted of seven subjects, Cluster II of two, Cluster III of six and Clusters IV and V each consisted of only one subject. For each of the five clusters, the neuropsychological variables were classified under the three following categories: left hemisphere, right hemisphere, and interhemispheric. To reveal the variability within a cluster and its relationship to the group mean, both the cluster mean and the individual scores for each stutterer are presented in Tables 4.2 and 4.3. Significant differences from a control population (Yeudall et al., 1986; Yeudall et al., 1987), matched by age, sex, handedness and Full Scale IQ, for both the group mean and individual scores of each stutterer are indicated by asterisks. The data were further summarized (see Table 4.6) regarding the functional integrity of the central nervous system for each stutterer as determined by the different assessment modalities.

Results

Cluster I

The first cluster (Table 4.2) consists of seven stutterers whose group mean shows, not unexpectedly, mild impairments for Oral Word Fluency (but not for the written equivalent of the test), name writing speed for both hands, and pegs placed using the right hand and both hands together for the Purdue Pegboard. As a group they show equal or better performance for most of the other variables compared to the controls. The two significant motor impairments for the right hand, along with Oral Word Fluency, would be consistent with compromised functioning of the more posterior frontal regions of the left hemisphere.

The finding that only one of the putative interhemispheric variables, Purdue Pegboard—both hands, was significant may be due to

Table 4.2   Mean and Individual Neuropsychological Scores for Clusters I and II

	Mean	S_1	S_2	S_3	S_4
					Cluster I
Left Hemisphere					
WCST:E	15.4	25.0	9.0	3.0	45.0*
WCST:S	5.3	6.0	6.0	6.0	1.0*
TPT:R	238.4	185.2	177.0	255.0	254.0
TMB	50.6	37.4	48.0	49.0	38.0
SD:W	55.6	60.0	54.0	60.0	51.0
SD:O	60.9	65.0	61.0	78.0	67.0
PP:R	13.6*	17.0	15.0	11.0*	10.0*
OWF	10.5*	16.0	6.0*	13.0	14.3
WWF	11.1	15.0	8.7*	12.0	13.3
NW:R	1.2*	.4	.5	.5	.5
FT:R	45.8	45.0	37.2*	39.4*	41.2*
D:R	49.7	27.5	63.0	49.0	39.2
Right Hemisphere					
HCT	38.1	40.0	30.0	27.0	18.0
TPT:L	163.6	162.2	166.0	128.0	214.0
SG	.5	.9	.4	.6	.5
TMA	23.9	17.3	21.0	25.0	26.0
PP:L	14.1	17.0	12.0*	13.0	15.0
NW:L	3.7*	.8	1.2	1.1	1.5
FT:L	42.3	47.8	31.0*	39.2*	38.8*
D:L	43.5	29.0	58.5	38.8	24.5*
Interhemispheric					
TPT:B	102.5	98.0	191.0*	65.0	63.0
PP:A	38.4	49.0	41.0	37.0	33.0*
PP:B	11.1*	15.0	10.0*	11.0*	9.0*
Demographic					
Age	28.7	28.0	26.0	38.0	19.0
FSIQ	114.8	99.0	ND	128.0	ND
VIQ	112.5	93.0	ND	117.0	ND
PIQ	115.8	110.0	ND	138.0	ND
V-PIQ	-3.3	-17.0	-	-21.0	-
Sex		F	M	M	M

* = 1 S.D. or greater (poorer performance) than the control means based on data matched for age, sex handedness and IQ
ND = Not Done

S_5	S_6	S_7		Cluster II	
			Mean	S_1	S_2
5.0	2.0	19.0	15.5	9.0	22.0
6.0	6.0	6.0	6.0	6.0	6.0
279.3	280.1	238.0	647.0*	701.0*	592.9*
45.8	73.4	62.5*	58.8	66.5*	51.0
50.0	53.0	61.0	45.0*	44.0*	46.0
33.0*	60.0	62.0*	52.0*	54.0*	50.0*
15.0	12.0*	15.0	14.5	13.0*	16.0
7.3*	10.7*	6.0*	9.5*	7.7*	11.3*
7.7*	12.3	8.7*	9.5*	8.3*	10.7*
.7	5.6*	.5	.5	.6*	.4
38.2*	62.4	57.2	48.9	42.6*	55.2
48.5	54.3	66.5	42.8	44.0	41.5*
56.0*	61.0*	35.0	18.0	15.0	21.0
110.0	184.9	180.0	367.0*	491.0*	242.9
.1	.7	.6	.1	.0*	.2*
20.5	32.7*	25.0	25.1	24.0	26.2
14.0	13.0	15.0	15.5	13.0*	18.0
2.3*	17.7*	1.4	1.2	1.6*	.7
36.4*	54.8	48.4	38.7*	33.4*	44.0
45.5	44.5	64.0	41.8	40.5	43.0
47.7	172.7	80.0	152.3	143.2	161.3
38.0	32.0*	39.0	35.0	36.0*	34.0*
10.0*	10.0*	13.0	10.5*	9.0*	12.0
18.0	48.0	24.0	30.0	17.0	43.0
104.0	128.0	ND	110.0	113.0	107.0
102.0	138.0	ND	110.0	106.0	114.0
105.0	110.0	ND	110.5	123.0	98.0
-3.0	+28.0	-	-0.5	-17.0	+16.0
M	M	M		M	M

Table 4.3   Mean and Individual Neuropsychological Scores for Clusters III, IV and V

	Mean	S_1	S_2	S_3	S_4
				Cluster III	
Left Hemisphere					
WCST:E	10.0	18.0	8.0	5.0	3.0
WCST:S	6.0	6.0	6.0	6.0	6.0
TPT:R	380.6	318.0	305.8	360.1	449.4*
TMB	64.9	92.5*	86.9*	55.5	39.4
SD:W	53.5	43.0*	48.0	48.0*	54.0
SD:O	48.0	24.0*	42.0*	51.0*	74.0
PP:R	14.3	12.0*	13.0*	15.0	16.0
OWF	9.5*	8.0*	4.3*	10.0*	15.7
WWF	11.3	8.3*	4.0*	10.7*	18.0
NW:R	5.7*	.7*	7.1*	7.3*	6.8*
FT:R	48.2	45.6	47.0	42.2	55.6
D:R		61.8	53.0	26.0	51.5
Right Hemisphere					
HCT	51.7	82.0*	54.0*	59.0*	63.0*
TPT:L	220.8	225.8	261.9	165.2	209.6
SG	.6	.1*	.5	.6	.4
TMA	26.0	37.2*	28.4	21.9	16.8
PP:L	13.8	12.0*	12.0*	14.0*	15.0
NW:L	5.2*	1.8	15.3*	28.8*	19.5*
FT:L	42.5	41.4	38.6*	39.4	54.8
D:L		53.8	49.5	20.3	50.3
Interhemispheric					
TPT:B	120.9	98.5	105.1	88.0	97.5
PP:A	38.8	29.0*	38.0	45.0	42.0
PP:B	11.8	9.0*	10.0*	13.0	14.0
Demographic					
Age	38.0	33.0	36.0	47.0	31.0
FSIQ	104.5	88.0	106.0	107.0	105.0
VIQ	100.7	88.0	106.0	97.0	101.0
PIQ	110.0	94.0	104.0	120.0	112.0
V-PIQ	-7.7	-6.0	+2.0	-13.0	-11.0
Sex		M	M	F	M

* = 1 S.D. or greater (poorer performance) than the control means based on data matched for age, sex handedness and IQ
ND = Not Done

S$_5$	S$_6$	Cluster IV S$_1$	Cluster V S$_1$
17.0	9.0	28.0	8.0
6.0	6.0	6.0	6.0
443.3*	406.9*	900.0*	244.0
49.2	65.9	118.7*	54.0
57.0	71.0	33.0*	51.0*
61.0	36.0*	26.0*	59.0
15.0	15.0	15.0	11.0*
10.7*	8.3*	9.7*	11.3*
13.3	13.7	13.0	12.3
5.5*	7.0*	5.5*	.6
45.0	53.8	36.4*	42.0*
26.8	24.5	26.8	37.3*
25.0	27.0	89.0*	25.0
181.3	280.8*	809.9*	529.0*
.9	1.0	.2*	.8
21.4	30.5	42.7*	36.0*
16.0	14.0*	14.0*	14.0
11.1*	14.8*	18.3*	1.5*
31.4*	49.6	35.2*	33.4*
25.8	19.5*	22.8*	34.0*
192.5	144.0	444.3*	158.0*
36.0	43.0	26.0*	41.0
12.0	13.0	11.0*	13.0
37.0	44.0	55.0	26.0
117.0	104.0	91.0	121.0
113.0	99.0	93.0	122.0
117.0	113.0	90.0	118.0
-4.0	-14.0	-7.0	+4.0
F	F	F	M

chance, or to the nature of the three tests in this category. That is, the both hands subtest of the Purdue Pegboard is a relatively simple perceptual motor task and is more likely associated with the integrity of the posterior premotor and motor regions of the brain. In contrast, the Tactual Performance Test and the assemblies subtest of the Purdue Pegboard are more complex in nature and consequently would be expected to involve the anterior premotor and prefrontal regions of the brain. Thus, the mean performance for these two tasks is consistent with the normal performance observed for the Halstead Category and Wisconsin Card Sorting Test, which are the most sensitive measures of the functional integrity of the prefrontal regions of the brain. The significantly slowed both hands performance for Purdue Pegboard does not appear to reflect interhemispheric interference, as this can be accounted for by the unilateral slowing of the right hand, thus implicating involvement of the left hemisphere. In summary, the group data for the variables of Cluster I implicate essentially normal functioning of the frontal brain regions, with the possibility of weaker or compromised functioning of the more posterior and inferior motor speech regions of the left hemisphere.

Examination of the individual neuropsychological performances of the stutterers comprising Cluster I reveals a great deal of variability. Excluding deficits for the two tasks dependent upon fluent speech (Oral Word Fluency and Symbol Digit: Oral), one of the 21 variables would be expected to be significant at the five percent level of chance. However, only one stutterer (S_1) shows one or less significant neuropsychological impairments when compared to matched normal controls. Six of the seven stutterers (85.7%) have a significant number of impairments with four (66.7%) implicating bilateral posterior involvement of the frontal lobes with a left-sided emphasis. The significantly slower group mean name writing speed for the left hand is primarily due to one stutterer (S_6) and does not reflect the general performance of the stutterers in this cluster. Of the five stutterers who show significantly reduced performance for the both hands subtest of the Purdue Pegboard, four have unilateral impairments, with three showing greater involvement of the right hand (S_3, S_4 and S_6). Their individual results, as well as the group mean, could be accounted for by a left hemisphere effect without evoking a hypothesis of interhemispheric interference. One stutterer (S_5), however, shows normal performance for the Purdue Pegboard right and left hand but significant impairment with both hands, a finding consistent with an interpretation of interhemispheric interference. Interhemispheric interference is also suggested by the performance of another stutterer (S_2), who shows a significantly poorer performance on the both hands trial of the Tactual Performance Test, while showing better than normal performance for the right and left hand. The intellectual level of the four stutterers assessed in Cluster I indicates above average intelligence for the overall group. Variability is evident not only for the Full Scale IQ, but for the Verbal minus Performance IQ difference. Of the three stutterers showing differences of greater than 15 IQ points, two have a lower Verbal IQ.

Five of the seven stutterers in Cluster I completed the standard brainstem evoked potential assessment (Table 4.4). Wave I could not be reliability identified for two of the stutterers (S_2 and S_3) nor could waves III and V for S_3. The group mean data reveal no significant interpeak latency differences. However, abnormal "shortened" interpeak latencies are observed in four of the five (80%) stutterers with complete data; with three of the four (S_1, S_4 and S_6) showing faster right brainstem latencies. One of the stutterers (S_2), who did not complete the standard assessment, shows abnormal responses under the stressor condition (Table 4.6). His right wave latency response during the stressor task is slightly faster than the left (L>R) and the latency shift (R=L) associated with the increased stimulus rate is significantly shorter than normal. Thus, of the five stutterers showing evidence of compromised brainstem functioning, four (S_1, S_2, S_4 and S_6) show shorter conduction time for the right side.

Two of the three stutterers (S_1 and S_5) who were administered the Galambos 40 Hz procedure show abnormal phase shifts over the posterior frontal region (F_7) of the left hemisphere (Table 4.6). This same site, as well as the left mid-temporal region (T_3), is abnormal for the MLR of the third stutterer (S_6). The abnormal middle latency responses implicate involvement of the left hemisphere, possibly of subcortical origin, in all of the stutterers tested in this cluster. The

Table 4.4   Mean and Individual Scores for Brainstem Auditory Evoked Potentials

				Cluster I	
	Mean[a]	S_1	S_2	S_3	S_4
R: I-III	2.02	2.04	2.04	IC	1.88
R: III-V	1.77	1.60	2.12	IC	1.76
R: I-V	3.79	3.64*	4.16	IC	3.64*
L: I-III	2.09	1.96	IC	2.34	2.22
L: III-V	1.91	1.89	1.92	1.86	1.90
L: I-V	4.00	3.85	IC	4.20	4.12
R-L: I-III	-.07	+.08	IC	IC	-.34
R-L: III-V	-.14	-.29	+.20	IC	-.14
R-L: I-V	-.21	-.21	IC	IC	-.48*

				Cluster III	
	Mean	S_1	S_2	S_3	S_4
R: I-III	2.14	2.24	2.05	2.16	1.76
R: III-V	1.97	2.18	2.22	1.62	1.86
R: I-V	4.10	4.42	4.27	3.78	3.62*
L: I-III	2.17	IC	2.12	2.20	2.05
L: III-V	1.87	2.02	2.11	1.36*	1.89
L: I-V	4.01	IC	4.23	3.56*	3.94
R-L: I-III	-.03	IC	-.07	-.04	-.29
R-L: III-V	+.10	+.16	+.11	+.26	-.03
R-L: I-V	+.03	IC	+.04	+.22	-.32

* = Shortened latency: 99% Confidence Limits (p = .95)

IC = Incomplete

[a] = Mean latency is based on 5S (S_1, S_4, S_5, S_6 & S_7) with complete data for left and right ear stimulation

| S_5 | S_6 | S_7 | Cluster II | | |
			Mean	S_1	S_2
1.96	1.94	2.30	2.11	2.12	2.10
1.80	1.83	1.86	1.98	1.88	2.08
3.76	3.77	4.16	4.09	4.00	4.18
1.96	2.11	2.20	2.29	2.20	2.38
1.60	2.07	2.10	2.14	1.98	2.30
3.56*	4.18	4.30	4.43	4.18	4.68
0.00	-.17	+.10	-.18	-.08	-.28
+.20	-.24	-.24	-.16	-.10	-.22
+.20	-.41*	-.14	-.34*	-.18	-.50*

| S_5 | S_6 | Cluster IV | Cluster V |
		S_1	S_1
2.40	2.20	1.91	1.94
2.00	1.92	1.71	2.04
4.40	4.12	3.62*	3.98
2.32	2.14	1.77	2.14
1.86	2.00	1.98	2.18
4.18	4.14	3.75	4.32
+.08	+.06	+.14	-.30
+.14	-.08	-.27	-.14
+.22	-.02	-.13	-.34*

qEEG findings indicate that four of the seven (57%) stutterers (S_1, S_2, S_6 and S_7) have abnormal R/L hemispheric coherency ratios, when compared to controls (Tables 4.5 and 4.6). Two stutterers (33%) during Oral Word Fluency show significantly less coherency with the most frequently observed abnormal R/L coherency comparisons equally involving the prefrontal (Fp_1), posterior frontal (F_7) and mid-temporal (T_3) regions of the left hemisphere. In contrast, two stutterers (29%) show significantly less coherency during the performance of the visual spatial task, with the prefrontal (Fp_2) region, followed by the mid-temporal region (T_4), being the most frequently involved regions of the right hemisphere.

Cluster II

Cluster II is comprised of two individuals who show a significant number of neuropsychological deficits (Table 4.2). The pattern of deficits implicates compromised functioning of the premotor regions of the left hemisphere in both cases, with one stutterer (S_1) showing significant bilateral involvement of the motor regions as well. As in Cluster I, both stutterers show normal performance on the two measures most sensitive to the functional integrity of the prefrontal regions of the brain (WCST, HCT). In contrast, these two individuals show more global impairments and greater compromised functioning of the left hemisphere as implicated by their right hand deficits for the Tactual Performance Test. Their impaired interhemispheric scores for the Purdue Pegboard, as in Cluster I, can be explained as a left hemisphere effect (poor right-hand performance). Again, as in Cluster I, the range of the Verbal-Performance IQ difference is of a similar magnitude, varying from -17.0 to +16.0 points.

Examination of Cluster II brainstem evoked potential group mean responses reveals normal left and right brainstem interpeak latencies. However, the right minus left I-V interpeak latency difference is abnormal, for one stutterer (S_2) with the right side showing the shorter latency (Table 4.4). Furthermore, under the stressor condition, the other stutterer shows a prolongation of wave V for the left brainstem, again implicating faster right brainstem activity (Table 4.6). Normal responses are observed for both middle latency procedures for the one stutterer assessed on these two measures. The qEEG findings are abnormal for one stutterer (S_2), who shows less coherency between the posterior frontal (F_7) and temporal (T_3) regions of the left hemisphere during the performance of the Oral Word Fluency task. Both stutterers show normal coherency values during the performance of the visual spatial task (Tables 4.5 and 4.6).

Cluster III

The mean neuropsychological performances of the six individuals in this cluster are essentially equal to or better than the normal controls, except for oral word fluency and name writing speed (Table 4.3). Examination of each individual's performance reveals a significant number of deficits for four of the stutterers (S_1, S_2, S_3 and S_5) which are averaged or washed out when the group means are calculated. Of interest, all six stutterers show significantly slower name writing speed for the right hand, and five for the left hand. For these four stutterers, involvement of the premotor regions is implicated with a left-sided emphasis. The individuals in this cluster, compared to Cluster I, clearly show more neuropsychological impairments, particularly implicating involvement of the premotor and motor regions, with four showing mild impairments implicating the prefrontal regions, most likely of the right hemisphere. Impairment in these prefrontal measures appears to be one of the major variables in differentiating Cluster III from II, whose two subjects also show a large number of significant neuropsychological impairments. Variability is evident, as in Cluster I and II, for the Verbal-Performance difference in IQ, with the three stutterers showing the largest deviations having lower Verbal IQ.

Brainstem auditory evoked potentials do not reveal any group mean differences from the controls (Table 4.4). Wave I for the left side could not be identified for one stutterer (S_1). Of the five stutterers who completed the brainstem assessment, two (S_3 and S_4) show shortened interpeak latencies. A third stutterer (S_1) shows a bilateral (R>L) delayed wave V absolute latency abnormality under the stress condition, with the shift condition revealing a significantly shortened latency difference for the left side (Table 4.6).

Table 4.5 Stutterers Alpha Normalized Left/Right Coherency Ratios for Oral Word Fluency and Block Design

Cluster	Ss	Fp_1F_7 / Fp_2F_8		Fp_1T_3 / Fp_2T_4	
		OWF	BD	OWF	BD
I	1*	0.97	0.94	0.12[e]	1.04
I	2	1.17	1.64[e]	1.37	2.89[e]
I	3	1.09	0.92	0.92	0.96
I	4	1.08	0.90	1.13	1.06
I	5	0.99	1.03	0.92	1.01
I	6	ND	1.31	ND	2.47[d]
I	7	0.65[d]	1.08	0.66[a]	0.96
II	1	0.91	0.77	0.79	0.65
II	2	0.87	0.98	1.83	1.03
III	1	0.91	ND	0.70[a]	ND
III	2	ND	1.08	ND	0.98
III	3*	ND	0.89	ND	2.30
III	4	0.33[e]	1.13	0.75	0.62
III	5*	ND	1.04	ND	1.01
III	6*	0.93	1.27[b]	1.08	2.19
IV	1*	0.92[a]	1.24[a]	0.81[a]	2.92[e]
V	1	1.30	1.15[a]	1.23	1.41
Controls					
Male		0.95	0.94	0.94	1.08
S.D.		0.12	0.21	0.23	0.49
Female		1.10	1.01	1.13	1.42
S.D.		0.18	0.17	0.32	1.04

[a] = ±1.0 to ±1.49 S.D. from control means
[b] = ±1.5 to ±1.99 S.D. from control means
[c] = ±2.0 to ±2.49 S.D. from control means
[d] = ±2.5 to ±2.99 S.D. from control means
[e] = ±3.0 or greater S.D. from control means
* = Female
ND = Not Done

F_7T_3 / F_8T_4		Fp_1P_3 / Fp_2P_4		F_7P_3 / F_8P_4	
OWF	BD	OWF	BD	OWF	BD
0.17[e]	1.47	0.72	0.85	0.71	0.88
1.61	1.27	0.76	0.52	0.91	0.62
1.10	1.04	1.02	0.97	1.07	1.16
1.51	0.90	0.83	0.70	1.03	0.70
0.91	1.06	0.98	1.18	0.93	1.12
ND	1.20	ND	1.85[c]	ND	1.34
2.44	0.99	1.35	0.93	3.77	1.24
0.91	1.31	0.85	0.76	1.01	0.68
0.46[c]	1.33	1.92	0.74	0.65	0.76
0.62[b]	ND	1.53	ND	0.99	ND
ND	1.03	ND	0.98	ND	1.27
ND	1.56	ND	0.87	ND	1.13
0.96	0.62	0.44[a]	0.97	1.20	0.85
ND	0.71	ND	0.55	ND	0.84
1.24	1.20	1.38	2.80[c]	1.94	3.88[e]
1.16	1.92	0.57[a]	2.38[b]	0.77	2.74[d]
1.91	2.21[e]	1.32	0.57	1.88	0.42
1.01	1.18	1.07	1.02	1.16	1.30
0.26	0.32	0.42	0.40	0.52	0.44
1.01	1.52	1.24	1.31	1.69	1.45
0.21	1.23	0.53	0.64	1.62	0.51

Table 4.6   Summary of Diagnostic Findings for All Stutterers Across Assessment Modalities

| Cluster | Ss | Brainstem Evoked Potentials | | | Thalamus/Cortex Middle Latencies | |
		IPLs	Limits	Shift	40 Hz	MLRs
I	1	Rc*	ND	ND	F7PS	Norm
I	2	IC	L>R+	R=L*	ND	ND
I	3	IC	Norm	Norm	ND	ND
I	4	Rc*	L+	R*	ND	ND
I	5	Lc*	ND	ND	F7PS	Norm
I	6	R*-Lc	ND	ND	Norm	F7T3A
I	7	Norm	Norm	Norm	ND	ND
II	1	Norm	L+	Norm	ND	ND
II	2	R*-Lc	ND	ND	Norm	Norm
III	1	IC	R>L+	L*	ND	ND
III	2	Norm	ND	ND	Norm	C3A
III	3	Lc*	ND	ND	T4PS	C3Cz
III	4	Rc*	ND	ND	Norm	F7C3A
III	5	Norm	ND	ND	C3DW	C3A
III	6	Norm	ND	ND	F7DW	C4A
IV	1	Rc*	ND	ND	T3DW	C3A
V	1	R*-Lc	Norm	Norm	ND	ND
Abnormal		64%	57%	43%	60%	70%

L = Left	a = I-III IPL
R = Right	b = III-V IPL
B = left equal right impairment	c = I-V IPL
R>L = right more iimpiared than left	R-L = right minus left IPL
L>R = left more impaired than right	differences
Norm = Normal	IC = incomplete, wave I not
ND = Not Done	identifiable

PF = prefrontal region
PM = premotor frontal region
PoF = posterior frontal region
IH = interhemisphere

Cortex Neuropsychology		Dynamic Brain Activity Abnormal qEEG R/L Coherency	
PoF&PM	PreF	OWF	BD
Norm	Norm	F_7-T_3,Fp_1-T_3	Norm
R>L	Norm	Norm	F_8-Fp_2,Fp_2-T_4
L	Norm	Norm	Norm
L>R	L	Norm	Norm
L>R	R	Norm	Norm
Norm	R	ND	Fp_2-T_4,Fp_2-P_4
L	Norm	F_7-Fp_1	Norm
L>R	Norm	Norm	Norm
L	Norm	F_7-T_3	Norm
L>R	R	F_7-T_3,Fp_1-T_3	Norm
L>R	R	ND	Norm
L>R	R	ND	Norm
Norm	R	Fp_1-F_7,Fp_1-P_3	Norm
L>R	Norm	ND	Norm
R>L	Norm	Norm	F_8-P_4,F_8-Fp_2, Fp_2-P_4
L>R	R	F_7-Fp_1,Fp_1-T_3, Fp_1-P_3	Fp_2-T_4,F_8-P_4, Fp_2-P_4,F_8-Fp_2
R>L	Norm	Norm	F_8-T_4,F_8-Fp_2
88.2%		46.2%	29.4%

Fp_1 = left prefrontal
F_7 = left posterior inferior frontal
T_3 = left mid-temporal
C_3 = left superior central
P_3 = left superior parietal
C_z = central references
Fp_2 = right prefrontal
F_8 = right posterior inferior frontal
T_4 = right mid-temporal
C_4 = right superior central
P_4 = right superior parietal

PS = phase shift
DW = disintegrated wave form
A = low amplitude

* = shortened latency
(99% confidence limits p<.05)
+ = delayed latency
(99% confidence limits p<.05)

Galambos 40 Hz procedure was completed for five of the six stutterers with three (60%) showing an abnormal response. The abnormality for two individuals (S_5 and S_6) involves the posterior motor regions (C_3 and F_7) of the left hemisphere and for the other (S_3), involves the temporal lobe (T_4) of the right hemisphere (Table 4.6). All five of the stutterers, administered the MLR, show abnormal responses with four (80%) having a reduced amplitude over the superior central motor region (C_3) of the left hemisphere. One of these Ss (S_4) also had abnormal response over the left posterior frontal region (F_7). The remaining individual (S_6) shows an abnormal MLR over the right central region (C_4). Of interest, this individual also shows a Galambos 40 Hz abnormality over the left posterior frontal region (F_7). Sufficient artifact-free data for the qEEG analysis during the performance of the Oral Word task was obtained from only three of the six stutterers. Two of the three (S_1 and S_4) show significantly reduced left hemisphere coherency, with the prefrontal region (Fp1) being more involved than the posterior frontal region (F_7). The third stutterer (S_6) shows significantly reduced right hemisphere coherency during the performance of the spatial task (Table 4.5 and 4.6).

Cluster IV

This cluster consists of one female stutterer who shows a significantly impaired neuropsychological profile (Table 4.3). The pattern of her deficits implicates moderate involvement of the right prefrontal and the premotor regions of both hemispheres. The severity of her bilateral motor impairments is also reflected by her significant impairments for all three interhemispheric variables. This stutterer shows an asymmetrical shortened right I-V interpeak latency for the right brainstem (Table 4.4) and abnormal MLR (C_3) and Galambos 40 Hz (T_3) responses of the left hemisphere (Table 4.6). The qEEG left/right coherency ratios during the oral word task were also abnormal over the left hemisphere; F_7-Fp_1, Fp_1-T_3 and Fp_1-P_3. Furthermore, reduced coherency of the right prefrontal region (Fp_2) were observed during the performance of the spatial task. This latter finding is consistent with the right prefrontal dysfunction implicated by her neuropsychological results. Thus, this female stutterer shows significant impairments for all of the assessment measures, with her neuropsychological impairments and qEEG abnormalities being greater than those of any other stutterer in the study. Of particular interest, she is the only stutterer who did not show typical gains after treatment with respect to reduction in percentage of stuttering (Table 4.7).

Cluster V

This cluster consists of one male stutterer whose neuropsychological impairments implicate bilateral involvement of the premotor and posterior frontal regions, with a right hemisphere emphasis (Table 4.3). A significant right minus left I-V interpeak brainstem latency asymmetry is also observed for this stutterer, with the right-side response being significantly faster (Table 4.4). The Galambos 40 Hz and MLR procedures were not performed on this subject. His qEEG findings for the Oral Word Fluency task are normal whereas he shows significantly reduced coherencies during the performance of the spatial task, with more involvement of the right posterior frontal region (F_8) (Tables 4.5 and 4.6).

Summary and Discussion

Cluster analysis of the 17 stutterers on the neuropsychological variables yields five clusters. The mean data of each cluster, when compared to fluent controls (N=50), indicates overall normal values for two of the five clusters (I and III) which represents 76.5% of the sample. However, examination of the individual neuropsychological data reveals a significant degree of abnormal inter-subject variability for both of these clusters. Comparison of each stutterer's performance with fluent controls implicates compromised functioning of the motor strip and premotor regions for five of the stutterers in Cluster I. In Cluster III, every stutterer has an abnormal neuropsychological profile. The individuals in Clusters I, II, IV and V show impairments primarily localized to the motor and premotor regions.

	Rate of Speech		Percentage of Stuttering	
Subjects	PRE-SPM	POST-SPM	PRE	POST
Cluster I				
Subject 1	ND	ND	ND	ND
Subject 2	ND	ND	ND	ND
Subject 3	182.90	192.90	3.30	0.37
Subject 4	140.40	138.10	9.83	0.59
Subject 5	28.20	149.60	52.45	0.00
Subject 6[a]	19.00	167.00	61.00	4.20
Subject 7	170.60	196.00	6.03	0.97
Cluster II				
Subject 1	69.03	157.20	32.20	3.00
Subject 2[a]	ND	ND	ND	ND
Cluster III				
Subject 1	13.00	142.30	67.20	5.60
Subject 2	66.00	85.00	42.50	15.40
Subject 3[a]	ND	ND	ND	ND
Subject 4	162.00	174.00	17.10	0.20
Subject 5	98.30	172.70	26.30	0.00
Subject 6[a]	ND	ND	ND	ND
Cluster IV	32.00	80.00	40.70	50.40
Cluster V	153.20	164.50	7.20	1.30

TABLE 4.7 Summary of Clinical Speech Data for all Stutterers Before and After a Three-Week Intensive Stuttering Clinic

[a] = Subject who did not participate in a three-week (Boberg-Kully) stuttering treatment program.
ND = Not Done

In contrast, four of the six stutterers in Cluster III also show mild impairments on tests sensitive to the prefrontal regions of the brain. The significant degree of variation and large number of significant impairments for individual stutterers are obscured by the group mean data in the two major clusters (I and III). Overall, 88.2% of the stutterers have significant neuropsychological impairments for measures which are considered to be sensitive to the functional integrity of the frontal lobes of the brain. The differentiation between premotor and posterior frontal involvement is based primarily on theoretical brain-behavior relationships. An anterior (prefrontal) versus posterior (motor regions) frontal lobe differentiation is more tenable based on the traditional interpretation of the neuropsychological variables. From this perspective, the abnormal scores implicate compromised functioning of the brain which is more consistently localized to the frontal motor systems, even in those cases for which there is some evidence implicating mild involvement of the prefrontal regions of the brain. In relation to those measures considered to be more sensitive to the motor regions of the frontal lobes, the majority of the stutterers show evidence of greater involvement of the left hemisphere.

The second noteworthy finding is the high incidence (64%) of brainstem abnormalities, for which 75% of the stutterers show an asymmetrical fast conduction time for the right side of the brainstem. Furthermore, of the seven stutterers who received a stressor condition, four (57%) have a delayed wave V abnormality, with two being left sided and two bilateral. Three of these stutterers also show a rate shift wave V latency difference abnormality for the stressor condition, with two having significantly shortened latencies compared to controls.

Another interesting finding is the number of significant abnormalities observed for the middle latency responses, which were obtained for 10 of the 17 stutterers in the study. Abnormal Galambos 40 Hz responses are observed in 60% of the cases, with five of six (83%) showing left sided involvement. The MLR is abnormal for 70% of the stutterers with the left side being involved in five cases (71.4%), the right side in one, and bilateral in the other. In contrast to the observed brainstem abnormalities, generalization of these findings is tentative, as only 10 of the of the 17 stutterers were assessed with the two middle latency procedures.

The qEEG findings reveal abnormal coherencies for 10 of the 17 stutterers (58.8%). Six of the 13 stutterers (46.2%) assessed during actual speech production show significantly reduced coherencies within the left hemisphere. The reduced coherencies involve the left posterior inferior frontal region (i.e., over Broca's region) in all six stutterers and the left anterior prefrontal region (Fp_1) in five of the cases. This left hemisphere effect is consistent with the results derived from the two middle latency procedures in which abnormalities over the left hemisphere are observed for 80% of the assessed cases. Five of the 17 stutterers (29.4%) assessed on the visual spatial tasks have significantly reduced right/left coherencies for the right hemisphere. The prefrontal (Fp_2) and the posterior inferior frontal region (F_8), in that order, are the two most frequently involved regions of the right hemisphere.

The stutterers assessed in this project were found to have a diversity of deficits implicating abnormalities at different levels of the central nervous system from the brainstem to the cerebral cortex. The data support the contention that there is a great deal of variability in the functional integrity of the central nervous system in stutterers. In a preliminary study, Boberg and Yeudall (1985) found variability in the neuropsychological profiles of four stutterers. Two controlled stutterers, who maintained their fluency over a period of many years, had essentially normal neuropsychological profiles, while two stutterers, who continually suffered from relapses, had abnormal neuropsychological profiles. Manz (1988) noted that three of the most neuropsychologically impaired stutterers in her study also experienced unusual difficulties in their treatment program, showed minimal progress in therapy and failed to reach their final target of normal speech rate. Based on these findings, she speculated that there may be subgroups within the population of stutterers that require different treatment strategies and that relapse rates may also be related to subgroups identifiable by means of neuropsychological variables. Similarly, in the present study, the four stutterers (S_1 in I,

S_1 and S_2 in III and S_1 in IV) who made the least gains in therapy showed a large number of significant neuropsychological deficits.

The neuropsychological findings of the present study implicate compromised functioning of the motor systems of the frontal lobes with a left-sided emphasis. Although neuropsychological measures sensitive to other regions of the brain were not employed in this study, the present findings are consistent with the hypothesis that stuttering behavior is correlated with compromised functional integrity of the cortical motor speech systems of the frontal lobes. The implication of greater involvement of the more anterior pre-frontal regions of the right hemisphere, in 50% of the stutterers, is consistent with previous findings and theoretical speculations as to the neuropsychological bases of stuttering behavior (Boberg et al., 1983; Yeudall, 1985). It is hypothesized that compromised functioning of the right hemisphere may place stutterers at higher risk for stuttering because of the disruptive effect of emotional functions, purportedly subserved by the right side of the brain. That is, compromised functioning of the right hemisphere would reduce the individual's ability to effectively modulate emotion (either positive or negative) and place them at greater risk for consequent disruption of fluent speech. This disruption of speech is further hypothesized to be the result of interference effects of the right hemisphere on the left hemisphere's functional executive control of the motor systems, both at cortical and subcortical levels of the brain, during speech production (Greiner et al., 1986; Yeudall, 1985).

The qEEG results also reveal significant variability in stutterers with five of the 13 who completed the verbal task showing only left hemisphere abnormalities during speech production, while three of 17 who completed the spatial task show only right hemisphere abnormalities. In contrast, only one stutterer was found to have bilateral abnormalities. However, it is possible that the four stutterers for whom valid data could not be obtained during speech production may have had bilateral involvement.

The large percentage of stutterers showing brainstem abnormalities (70.6%), when both the standard analysis and the stressor condition measures are combined, with 75% showing shorter right brainstem interpeak latencies, is consistent with earlier findings in smaller samples (Boberg et al., 1983; Yeudall, 1985). The faster latencies of the right brainstem in stutterers may reflect compromised functioning of their left brainstem. That is, shortened brainstem interpeak latencies could be due to a failure of normal interhemispheric inhibition or interaction at the level of the brainstem. Wada and Star (1983a; 1983b), in two elegant experiments, isolated the two sides of the brainstem by injecting Procaine HCL into the midline of the trapezoid body in cats (i.e., a reversible split brain preparation) or by surgically sectioning the trapezoid body in guinea pigs (i.e., an irreversible split brain preparation). They demonstrated that ipsilateral interpeak latencies for the auditory evoked brainstem response are a function of the dynamic interaction of the two sides of the brainstem. In both experiments they found that disconnection of the right from left brainstem, at the level of the trapezoid body, resulted in shortened ipsilateral latencies. This was a consequence of wave III disappearing, while wave IV (wave V in humans) occurred earlier. Since the ipsilateral auditory tract fibres had not been disturbed, the disappearance of wave III and the shortening of the I-IV interpeak latency on the same side of the brain being stimulated, can only be accounted for by the disconnection of one side from the influences of the other side of the brainstem. Thus, it appears that a shortened latency on one side of the brainstem may be due to a loss or reduction of the normal contralateral inhibitory effects of the other side of the brainstem. It follows from their findings, that the high incidence of shortened interpeak latencies for the right brainstem, observed in the stutterers in the present study, may be due to a failure in the normal inhibitory function of the left brainstem during speech production. If indeed this is the case, then the abnormal brainstem findings would be congruent with the evidence for left-sided abnormalities rostral to the level of the brainstem involving the thalamus and cortex as implicated by the middle latency, neuropsychological and qEEG findings in the present study.

Abnormal brainstem functioning has previously been reported by Blood and Blood (1984) in four moderate and four severe adult stutterers. In contrast to the present findings, they showed prolonged rather than shortened interpeak latencies in five of their eight cases, with three being bilateral and two right-sided. Examination of their data, in terms of right minus left interpeak latency differences (I-III, III-V and I-V), suggests that: three of their stutterers had relatively shortened latencies on the right side; one had shortened latencies bilaterally; one had bilaterally delayed latencies; one had delayed latencies for the left and another for the right side; one had a faster right I-III latency difference; and one had a delayed III-V latency difference. The high incidence of brainstem abnormalities in the present study, in conjunction with the findings of Blood and Blood (1984) and the findings reviewed by Rosenfield and Jerger (1984), is consistent with the emerging evidence for abnormalities of the auditory system at the level of the brainstem, at least in some stutterers. As previously suggested (Yeudall, 1985), stuttering behavior for many individuals may be a failure in the initiation of expiration associated with speech, which appears to be under control of the brainstem and midbrain/thalamic regions of the left hemisphere. The evidence, based on brainstem evoked potentials, is of importance because of its robust nature in terms of validity and near invariant reliability, compared to the variance associated with behavioral techniques (Hannley and Dorman, 1982).

Evidence for greater subcortical involvement of the left hemisphere is implicated by the two middle latency procedures. These measures reveal abnormalities in nine of the ten stutterers assessed (7 unilateral and 2 bilateral), with the left side being abnormal in all cases. These findings are supportive of the hypothesis of thalamic/subcortical involvement in stuttering behavior (Yeudall, 1985). The abnormal MLR over the superior central regions in five of the stutterers in the present study may be reflecting abnormal activity of the supplementary motor area (SMA) of the brain. As suggested by others (Webster, 1987; Yeudall, 1985), the failure of normal initiation of speech could occur at higher levels involving the midbrain/thalamic regions and the supplementary motor regions of the brain. Webster (1986) found that stutterers performing a sequential motor task could finger tap as fast as fluent speakers but achieved fewer sequential patterns, made more errors and had slower response initiation times.

Webster (1987) and Yeudall (1985) proposed that compromised functioning of the supplementary motor area may play a role in stuttering behavior because of its purported involvement in the initiation and modulation of speech and nonspeech sequential motor behavior (Damasio and Van Hoesen, 1980; Goldberg, 1985).

In conclusion, the results of this study implicate compromised functioning of the cortical motor regions of the two hemispheres (left greater than right) and left midbrain region in stutterers. Involvement of the left side of the brain may also exist at the level of the brainstem, if right shortened brainstem interpeak latencies reflect failure of left brainstem inhibition, as suggested by the studies of Wada and Starr (1983a, 1983b). Interhemispheric interference by the right hemisphere is a plausible hypothesis for the data observed in some of our stutterers. However, the data from the majority of stutterers in this study provide evidence of a fundamental disturbance of the left hemisphere motor systems. The use of a multidimensional assessment strategy to assess the functional integrity of the brain, at various levels, has provided evidence for a neurological substrate in the etiology of stuttering behavior, and a possible basis for a major source of variability in stutterers.

Acknowledgements

The senior author wishes to thank Dr. D. Brown for providing the evoked potential data from his laboratory, Jim Morrison and Vijaey Sangar for their technical assistance and Sharon Burkin for her assistance with the manuscript. The research was supported by the Austin S. Nelson Foundation, The Institute for Stuttering Treatment and Research, and Alberta Hospital Edmonton Research Committee.

References

Annett, M.A. (1970). A classification of hand preference by association analysis. *British Journal of Psychology* 61: 303–20.
Blood, I.M. and Blood, G.W. (1984). Relationship between stuttering severity

and brainstem-evoked response testing. *Perceptual and Motor Skills* 59: 935–38.

Boberg, E. and Kully, D. (1985). *Comprehensive Stuttering Program*. San Diego: College-Hill Press.

Boberg, E. and Yeudall, L.T. (1985). Clinical successes and failures in stuttering therapy: Some possible relationships to CNS functions. Research Bulletin #107, Alberta Hospital Edmonton.

Boberg, E., Yeudall, L.T., Schopflocher, D. and Bo-Lassen, P. (1983). The effect of an intensive behavioral program on the distribution of the distribution of EEG alpha power in stutterers during the processing of verbal and visuospatial information. *Journal of Fluency Disorder* 8: 245–63.

Brillinger, D.R. (1981). *Time Series*. San Francisco: Holden-Day.

Crosson, B. and Hughes, C.W. (1987). Role of the thalamus in language: Is it related to schizophrenic thought disorder? *Schizophrenia Bulletin* 13(4): 605–21.

Damasio, A. R., and VanHoesen, G.W. (1980). Structure and function of the supplementary motor area. *Neurology* 30: 359.

Fedora, O., Yeudall, L.T. and Lind, J. (1987). Brainstem auditory evoked potential control data. Research Bulletin #153, Department of Neuropsychology, Alberta Hospital Edmonton.

Galambos, R., Makeig, S. and Talmachoff, P.J. (1981). A 40-Hz auditory potential recorded from the human scalp. *Proceedings of the National Academy of Science* (Wash.) 78: 2643–47.

Goldberg, G. (1985). Supplementary motor area structure and function: review and hypotheses. *The Behavioral and Brain Sciences* 8: 567–616.

Gotman, J. (1987). Interhemispheric interactions in seizures of focal onset: data from human intracranial recordings. *Electroencephalography and Clinical Neurophysiology* 67: 120–33.

Greiner, J.R., Fitzgerald, H.E. and Cooke, P.A. (1986). Bimanual hand writing in right-handed and left-handed stutterers and nonstutterers. *Neuropsychologia* 24(3): 441–47.

Hall, J.W. and Jerger, J. (1978). Central auditory function in stutterers. *Journal of Speech and Hearing Research* 21: 324–37.

Hannley, M. and Dorman, M.F. (1982). Some observations on auditory function and stuttering. *Journal of Fluency Disorders* 7: 93–108.

Kraus, N., Ozdamar, O., Hier, D. and Stein, L. (1982). Auditory middle latency responses (MLRs) in patients with cortical lesions. *Electroencephalography and Clinical Neurophysiology* 54: 275–87.

Kraus, N., Smith, D.I. and McGee, T. (1988). Midline and temporal lobe MLRs in the guinea pig originate from different generator systems: A conceptual framework for new and existing data. *Electroencephalography and Clinical Neurophysiology* 70: 541–58.

Lasky, R.E. (1984). A developmental study on the effect of stimulus rate on the auditory evoked brain-stem response. *Electroencephalography and Clinical Neurophysiology* 59: 411–19.

Lieb, J.B., Hozue, K., Skomer, C.E. and Song, X.W. (1987). Interhemispheric propagation of human mesial temporal lobe seizures: A coherence/ phase analysis. *Electroencephalography and Clinical Neurophysiology* 67: 101–19.

Manz, L. (1988). "Clinical and neuropsychological measures as predictors of male stutterers' response to intensive stuttering therapy." Master's thesis, University of Alberta, Edmonton, Alberta.

Picton, T.W., Hilliyard, S.A. and Krausz, H.I. (1974). Human auditory evoked potentials. I. Evaluation of components. *Electroencephalography and Clinical Neurophysiology* 36: 179–90.

Pockberger, H., Petsche, H., Rappelsberger, P., Zidek, B. and Zapotoczky, H.G. (1985). On-Going EEG in Depression: A Topographic Spectral Analytical Pilot Study. *Electroencephalography and Clinical Neurophysiology* 61: 349–58.

Rosenfield, D.B. and Jerger, J. (1984). Stuttering and auditory function. In R.F. Curlee and W.H. Perkins, eds., *Nature and Treatment of Stuttering: New directions*, pp. 73–87. San Diego: College-Hill Press.

Rosenfield, D.B. and Nudelman, H.B. (1987). Neuropsychological models of speech dysfluency. In L. Rustin, H. Purser and D. Rowley, eds., *Progress in the Treatment of Fluency Disorders*, London: Taylor and Francis.

Royce, J.R., Yeudall, L.T. and Bock, C. (1976). Factor analytic studies of human brain damage: I. First and second-order factors and their brain correlates. *Multivariate Behavioral Research* 4: 381–418.

Spydell, J.D., Pattee, G. and Goldie, W.D. (1985). The 40 Hz event-related potential: Normal values and effects of lesions. *Electroencephalography and Clinical Neurophysiology* 62: 193–202.

Wada, S.I. and Starr, A. (1983a). Generation of auditory brain stem responses (ABRs). I. Effects of injection of a local anesthetic (procaine HCl) into the trapezoid body of guinea pigs and cat. *Electroencephalography and Clinical Neurophysiology* 56: 326–39.

———. (1983b). Generation of auditory brain stem responses (ABRs). II. Effects of surgical section of the trapezoid body on the ABR in guinea pigs and cat. *Electroencephalography and Clinical Neurophysiology* 56: 340–51.

Ward, J.H. (1963). Hierarchical grouping to optimize an objective function. *Journal of American Statistical Association* 58: 236–44.

Webster, W.G. (1986). Response sequence organization and reproduction by stutterers. *Neuropsychologia* 24(6): 813–21.

———. (1987). What hurried hands reveal about "Tangled Tongues": A neuropsychological approach to understanding stuttering. *Human Communication Canada* 11(3): 11–18.

Woods, D.L., Clayworth, C.C., Knight, R.T., Simpson, G.V. and Naeser, M.A. (1987). Generators of middle- and long-latency auditory evoked potentials: Implications of patients with bitemporal lesions. *Electroencephalography and Clinical Neurophysiology* 68: 132–48.

Yeudall, L.T. (1985). A neuropsychological theory of stuttering. In E. Boberg, ed., *Seminars in Speech and Language, Vol. III, Stuttering: Experimental Programs in Research*. New York: Thieme-Stratton.

Yeudall, L.T., Fromm, D., Reddon, J.R. and Stefanyk, W.O. (1986). Normative data stratified by age and sex for 12 neuropsychological tests. *Journal of Clinical Psychology* 42(6): 918–46.

Yeudall, L.T., Reddon, J.R., Gill, D.M. and Stefanyk, W.O. (1987). Normative data for the Halstead-Reitan neuropsychological test stratified by age and sex. *Journal of Clinical Psychology* 43: 346–67.

Zimmerman, G. (1984). Articulatory Dynamics of Stutterers. In R. Curlee and W. Perkins, eds., *Nature and Treatment of Stuttering: New Directions*. San Diego: College-Hill Press.

Editor's Note

This paper was submitted after the conference for publication in this book. There is no discussion section.

Richard F. Curlee

5 Neuropsychological Aspects of Stuttering
Implications for Diagnosis

As our understanding of the brain mechanisms responsible for normal speech and language and their disruption increases, so will our understanding of stuttering. Such advances could also lead to substantial improvements in the clinical management of stutterers. How can the findings from these areas of research be usefully applied at present to the diagnosis of stuttering?

Much of this research has compared the skills, abilities or functions of stutterers with those of nonstutterers or has contrasted such variables within stutterers during periods of speech judged to be stuttered with those judged to be free of stuttering. Such designs may provide interesting descriptive data, but they cannot support causal inferences. One cannot determine from these studies how those variables that covary are functionally related; which is the cause, which is the effect, or if, in fact, their concurrent changes merely reflect the effect of some other underlying, unobserved variable.

Even though a great deal of data on stutterers and on stuttering has been accumulated over the years, few testable accounts of the psychobiological mechanisms responsible for stuttering have been advanced to date. Moreover, it should be acknowledged that an accurate account of how such mechanisms result in stuttering may not necessarily lead to major changes in how stutterers are diagnosed or treated. Advances in understanding of disease processes usually improve the medical management of those diseases through their prevention; however, a number of abnormal conditions and chronic health problems continue to be managed symptomatically when prevention efforts are not successful. Thus, some information may not produce substantial changes in current diagnostic or treatment procedures.

Much of the physiological and neuropsychological information that has been presented in this book was obtained from adults. Adult stutterers consist of less than half of all those who ever stutter and should, therefore, be considered a functionally distinct subgroup of stutterers. The possibility that findings obtained from adults whose stuttering problems have persisted may not be pertinent to either the onset of stuttering or to its remission. Indeed, it has been suggested that such information may primarily depict characteristics that lead to or result from chronic stuttering (Andrews et al., 1983; Curlee, 1984). Thus, particular caution should be exercised in speculating about the application of such findings to children who stutter, or to their diagnosis and treatment.

Traditionally, most clinicians have dealt with stuttering as a perceptual phenomenon. Indeed, the diagnosis and treatment of most speech impairments are founded on perceptual evaluations and analyses. Probably the most widely used definition of stuttering is that proposed by Wingate (1964) who described it as a disruption in the fluency of speech that is characterized by involuntary, audible or silent, repetitions or prolongations of sounds, syllables and one-syllable words. He also noted that such disruptions usually occur frequently, are distinctive in appearance and are not readily controllable. For Wingate, these observable speech behaviors are obligatory manifestations, or the necessary and sufficient signs, of stuttering. The appearance of speech-related struggle or reports of negative emotional reactions are designated as accessory and associated features, respectively. This view of stuttering relies on human observers as the ultimate stuttering detection and measurement device (Young, 1984). Although neuropsychological and physiological accounts of stuttering and fluency are not incompatible with this view, some paradoxical interpretations of physiological data seem to have resulted.

For example, physiological events often do not correlate tidily with perceptions of fluent or dysfluent speech. The electromyographic (EMG) studies of Freeman and Ushijima (1978) and Shapiro (1980) found heightened, mistimed, nonreciprocal activity among laryngeal and, to a lesser extent, articulator muscle antagonists during segments of speech perceived as stuttered. Moreover, they also observed the same kinds of anomalous activity during some of the perceptually fluent speech segments of both stuttering and nonstuttering speakers, as well as apparently normal EMG activity during some perceived stutterings. As a consequence of these and others' findings, such terms as "sub-clinical" or "physiological" stuttering have been introduced to describe speech that does not sound dysfluent to listeners but evidences "abnormal" appearing electrophysiological tracings. It may be only a matter of time until some speech disruptions are characterized as "physiologically normal" stutterings. Such semantic paradoxes are bothersome and may add more than a little confusion to the literature.

W. Perkins (1983; 1984) attempted to focus attention on stuttering as a speech production event rather than a perceptual event. He views stuttering as an involuntary disruption of a speaker's continuing attempt to complete an utterance whose execution has already begun, an event which may or may not result in the perceptual events described by Wingate (1964). This view attempts to define stuttering in terms of events that occur as part of the production of stuttered speech but sees the acoustic signatures that are perceived by listeners as instances of stuttering as neither necessary nor sufficient evidence that stuttering has, in fact, occurred. Perkins argues that perceptual conceptualizations of stuttering have hampered progress toward a scientific understanding of its nature, and his views seem intuitively compatible with much of the research that has been described at this conference. Even though the idea that stuttering involves a speaker's momentary inability to complete an intended utterance is not new, nor widely disputed, its clinical and theoretical usefulness has not yet been demonstrated.

Medical diagnoses consist of identifying a disease from its signs and symptoms. In speech-language pathology, diagnoses typically involve analyzing the nature and severity of a problem from case history information, clinical examinations and observation, and standardized testing. Once stuttering has become severe or has been a chronic problem for some period of time, accurate diagnosis is seldom a problem, and most children who stutter can be readily distinguished from nonstuttering children, even those who are highly disfluent (Westby, 1979). Thus, there is a pattern of behavioral signs and symptoms that can usually be obtained from the case history or from observations that point unequivocally to a diagnosis of stuttering.

Diagnostic protocols for evaluating children who are suspected of incipient stuttering have been published (Adams, 1977; Curlee, 1980; Gregory and Hill, 1980; Pindzola and White, 1986). The similarities among these published protocols suggest that there is substantial agreement on how best to identify children who are beginning to stutter. Nevertheless, the speech of some children who are just beginning to stutter sounds much like that of other children their age much of the time. Their stuttering is so inconsistent and episodic, that few, if any, signs of stuttering may be observed during a formal evaluation. Under these circumstances, accurate identification of an incipient stutterer can be challenging for even an experienced clinician. It would be with these children that neuropsychological findings might prove to be most useful.

To what extent might neuropsychological testing be of assistance in identifying an incipient stutterer? Since currently available information has been obtained largely from chronic adult stutterers it cannot be applied to young children who stutter. In addition, this type of information characterizes the performance of groups of stutterers whose individual scores overlap with those of nonstutterers. As a consequence, even if comparable data were now available for preschool age stutterers and nonstutterers, and they are not, the overlap in the performance of the two groups would likely limit the diagnostic utility of such information. For example, it is well known that boys are much more likely to stutter than girls and that the offspring of stutterers are much more likely to stutter than are the stutterer's own siblings (Kidd, 1984). However, this information is of minimal value in trying to determine if a preschool girl, who has no first-degree stuttering relatives, is beginning to stutter. And this is precisely what needs to be determined. Would adding neuropsychological test findings to case history information and behavioral observations yield more accurate diagnoses of incipient stuttering? That is an empirical question that should be investigated. Additional research is needed before neuropsychological testing may be useful in differentiating incipient stutterers from their nonstuttering peers.

Perhaps neuropsychological testing holds more immediate promise for contributing to the case-selection decisions that result from diagnostic evaluations. Current evidence suggests that environmental factors, and each stutterer's idiosyncratic response to such factors, likely determine whether or not stuttering will persist, and if it does, how severe a problem it will be. There is substantial evidence that most children who begin to stutter stop, with or without receiving professional help, and that remission rates may be highest during the year following stuttering onset (Andrews, 1984). It is also known that remission of stuttering is inversely related to age and to the severity of the problem; that residual stuttering episodes are common for those whose remissions occur after adolescence; and that relapses after treatment are common among chronic adult stutterers (Bloodstein, 1987). This kind of information is of little help in deciding how long one should wait before intervening with a specific child, and as a result, such decisions currently rely on the judgement and expertise of individual clinicians. It is tempting to speculate, therefore, that some of the neuropsychological and physiological findings discussed in this book by Webster, Moore and Mateer may signal the development of chronic stuttering problems and could provide clinicians with a sounder basis for initiating or delaying treatment.

For example, Dr. Mateer (see Chapter 1) has indicated that stuttering probably involves some language functions or processes. It is known that phonological and language-learning problems are relatively common among school-age stutterers (Blood and Seider, 1981), and as Dr. Mateer noted, there is extensive anatomical overlap of motor speech and speech perception sites with anterior and posterior language sites, at least among nonstutterers. Similarly, Dr. Moore's research (see Chapter 2) has found that adult stutterers process linguistic stimuli with diminished activation of their left hemispheres, and he believes that they should profit from language training. These views provide some promising leads for future research and suggest that neurolinguistic functions may be involved in the onset or persistence of at least some stutterers' problems. Certainly, careful clinical assessment of young stutterers' language skills should be one component of their diagnostic evaluation.

In contrast, Dr. Webster has hypothesized that stuttering is symptomatic of a more general motor planning/sequencing/processing disorder rather than a speech disorder. He speculates that a "fragile supplementary motor area" in the left hemisphere may be disrupted by concurrent right hemisphere activity among stutterers and that this condition is irreversible, at least among adult stutterers. Perhaps young children who stop stuttering do not evidence this more general motor disorder or perhaps it resolves through maturation or treatment in contrast to those for whom stuttering does persist. This suggests that age-appropriate concurrent motor tasks might indicate which young stutterers are most likely to become chronic adult stutterers. Again, more study is needed.

On a related issue, Dr. Mateer also commented that early, diffuse brain damage may result in bilateral cerebral organization of speech-language functions and that larger than expected proportions of adult stutterers have been found to evidence such organization. This is consistent with Andrews et al. (1983) conclusion that early brain damage increases one's risk for becoming a stutterer and with the recent findings of Andrews et al. (1991) that the second-born twin is ordinarily the one who stutters in monozygotic twin pairs that are discordant for stuttering. Careful prospective studies of young children whose perinatal records indicate a high-risk of brain damage could provide additional insight on this issue.

These examples illustrate just a few of the possible clinical applications that might be explored through further systematic research with children who stutter. There are relatively few empirical studies of children who stutter, especially of those who stop stuttering. And even though important advances in our understanding of CNS functions have been made in recent years, the findings have not been integrated into a useful model or theory of stuttering. Consequently, the neuropsychological and physiological research on stuttering does not yet provide an adequate empirical or conceptual foundation on which to base diagnostic procedures with young stutterers. Because this research has been conducted largely with adults, it is reasonable to assume that it should be more pertinent to the diagnostic evaluations of adult stutterers.

Diagnostic evaluations of the fluency problems of adolescents and adults differ substantially from those with young children, but since the 1960s, little formal or systematic attention has been given clinically to either the etiology of stuttering or to its hypothesized underlying mechanisms. During this period, many programs came to rely on a variety of operant techniques for decreasing the frequency of stuttering, and clinical assessments came to emphasize the quantification of stutterers' problems, perhaps only by counting the frequency of his or her speech disruptions. Asking older children and adults a few case-history questions ordinarily elicited reports of a variety of symptoms that are common to stuttering and the opportunity to observe one or more of Wingate's (1964) obligatory signs of stuttering. Thus, an unequivocal diagnosis of stuttering can usually be established without difficulty from case history reports and behavioral observations, and the remainder of the diagnostic workup can be devoted to gathering data that are pertinent to assessing the severity and scope of stutterer's problem. While there is little apparent need to obtain other kinds of information (i.e., neuropsychological) in order to identify the existence of such problems in adults, few diagnostic evaluations are likely to be restricted to problem identification.

Most diagnostic evaluations of chronic adult stutterers likely include an assessment of both speaking and dysfluency rates during several speaking tasks and situations that can be used later as benchmarks with which to compare the clients' performance periodically during and after treatment. Some clinicians may also attempt to assess the naturalness of stutterers' speech, to sample some of their more severe speech disruptions, or to obtain measures of avoidance reactions, speech attitudes, anxiety, locus of control or other attributes that the clinician believes may be useful in planning treatment or in predicting clients' success in therapy. Some clinicians also report using interviews or paper and pencil tests to screen-out prospective stuttering clients whose concurrent health or psychiatric problems might complicate clinical management. Such assessment practices rely on traditional clinical techniques, and little, if any, attention is ordinarily directed to the physiological and neuropsychological variables that have been the focus of this conference. Some of these variables, however, could prove to be valuable prognostic indicators for adult stutterers.

Several current treatment practices appear to improve many stutterers' skills in reducing the frequency of perceptible disruptions of their speech, but such skills are not maintained, ordinarily, without a substantial amount of practice, vigilance and attention. Controlled stutter-free speech, when it is achieved, appears to be a performance, a skill that has been improved, rather than a competence that is acquired. Among adults, the biological machinery of the brain seems rarely able to reorganize or reprogram its functions so that stuttering ceases to be at least an occasional problem. Still, the treatment outcomes of some adult stutterers are clearly superior to those of others, even to a casual observer. Perhaps these differences in treatment outcomes may be related to some of the neuropsychological and physiological characteristics that have been discussed here, and in some way may index stutterers' capacities for improving fluency skills or the extent to which such skills have been acquired at termination of therapy.

Andrews and Craig (1988) recently reported, for example, that absence of any stuttering during speech assessment at the end of treatment, normalized S-24 scores, and improved (>10%) internalized locus of control scores predicted stutterers' maintenance of treatment gains. Dr. Webster (see Chapter 3) described stutterers' performance deficits during dual motor tasks which he has interpreted as reflecting the effects of interhemispheric interference. If such performance deficits model the types of brain functions or disruptions that result in stuttering, one might expect a stutterer's dual motor task abilities to reflect his capacity for meeting the neurophysiological demands for fluency and predict his potential for improving his speech through training. Dr. Moore has concluded that severe stutterers use fewer cognitive strategies in processing linguistic information, as shown by diminished left hemisphere activity during the performance of such tasks, than do mild stutterers or nonstutterers. The functional connections, if any, between such electrophysiological events and disrupted speech events have yet to be demonstrated, and their significance is not yet well understood. Nevertheless, hemispheric activation patterns may have prognostic value for adult stutterers prior to treatment or may predict either relapse or permanence of treatment effects after treatment. Careful, longitudinal study of even a few adult stutterers could indicate whether or not any of these possibilities may have useful clinical applications.

Clinical practices should be founded on empirical studies of the clinical utility and effectiveness of assessment and/or treatment procedures. The use of poorly understood research findings in the treatment of incipient or chronic stutterers may reflect well-intended hopes for dramatic clinical improvement, but responsible clinical practice should be based on conceptual understandings and controlled observations of the application of that understanding to clinical problems. At present, it seems clear to me that it is premature to apply the evidence that has been obtained to date from physiological and neuropsychological investigations of stutterers to the clinical diagnoses of either children or adults who stutter. This does not mean that such research will not have important clinical applications at some time in the future. It may. Only further study will tell.

Many current accounts of stuttering, such as those of Neilson and Neilson (1987) and Starkweather (1987) as well as Moore (Chapter 2), and Webster (Chapter 3), suggest that stutterers neurophysiological processing capacities are not sufficient to produce speech that is free of stuttering much of the time. The nature of the hypothesized diminished capacities and how stuttering results from them differs from account to account, but there appears to be an implicit consensus that a capacity-demands model is a fruitful vantage point from which to view the physiological and neuropsychological aspects of stuttering. It will be interesting to follow the evolution of these models in the future and how the underlying mechanisms of hypothesized capacities and demands are specified for empirical study.

Research and scientific inquiry often generate more questions than answers. For example, what specific endogeneous capacities predispose one to become a stutterer? How are these capacities compromised by such exogeneous factors as brain damage? What specific environmental demands contribute to the onset of stuttering problems? What specific capacities and demands lead to its persistence or to its remission? Do stuttered speech disruptions differ from nonstuttered speech disruptions, and if so, how does the speech production process of each differ? What demands precipitate the initiation of instances of stuttering? What capacities (mechanisms) permit the termination of such disruptions and the resumption of speech? What determines the topography of stuttering? These and other unanswered questions, as well as a number of unquestioned answers and beliefs about stuttering, need further critical study. Perhaps some key unasked questions are yet to be formulated. Nevertheless, there is reason to believe that we may be at the threshold of some major conceptual breakthroughs in our understanding of speech motor processing and of stuttering.

References

Adams, M. (1977). A clinical strategy for differentiating the normally nonfluent child and the incipient stutterer. *Journal of Fluency Disorders* 2: 141–48.

Andrews, G. (1984). Epidemiology of stuttering. In R. Curlee and W. Perkins, eds., *Nature and Treatment of Stuttering: New Directions*. San Diego: College-Hill Press.

Andrews, G. and Craig, A. (1988). Prediction of outcome after treatment for stuttering. *British Journal of Psychiatry* 153: 236–40.

Andrews, G., Craig, A., Feyer, A.M., Hoddinott, S., Howie, P. and Neilson, M. (1983). Stuttering: A review of research findings and theories circa 1982. *Journal of Speech and Hearing Disorders* 48: 226–46.

Andrews, G., Morris-Yates, A., Howie, P. and Martin, N.G. (1991). Genetic factors in stuttering confirmed. *Archives of General Psychiatry* 48: 1034–35

Blood, G. and Seider, R. (1981). The concomitant problems of young stutterers. *Journal of Speech and Hearing Disorders* 46: 31–33.

Bloodstein, O. (1987). *A handbook on stuttering* (4th ed.). Chicago: National Easter Seal Society.

Curlee, R. (1980). A case selection strategy for young disfluent children. *Seminars in Speech, Language and Hearing* 1: 277–87.

———. (1984). Stuttering disorders: An overview. In J. Costello, ed., *Speech Disorders in Children: Recent Advances*. San Diego: College-Hill Press.

Freeman, F. and Ushijima, T. (1978). Laryngeal muscle activity during stuttering. *Journal of Speech and Hearing Research* 21: 538–62.

Gregory, H. and Hill, D. (1980). Stuttering therapy for children. *Seminars in Speech, Language and Hearing* 1: 351–63

Kidd, K. (1984). Stuttering as a genetic disorder. In R. Curlee and W. Perkins, eds., *Nature and Treatment of Stuttering: New Directions*. San Diego: College-Hill Press.

Neilson, M. and Neilson, P. (1987). Speech motor control and stuttering: A computational model of adaptive sensory-motor processing. *Speech Communication* 6: 325–33.

Perkins, W. (1983). The problem of definition: Commentary on "Stuttering." *Journal of Speech and Hearing Disorders* 48: 246–49.

———. (1984). Stuttering as a categorical event: Barking up the wrong tree. *Journal of Speech and Hearing Disorders* 49: 431–34.

Pindzola, R. and White, D. (1986). A protocol for differentiating the incipient stutterer. *Language, Speech and Hearing Services in Schools* 17: 2–15.

Shapiro, A. (1980). An electromyographic analysis of the fluent and disfluent utterance of several types of stutterers. *Journal of Fluency Disorders* 5: 203–31.

Starkweather, C.W. (1987). *Fluency and Stuttering*. Englewood Cliffs, NJ: Prentice-Hall, Inc.

Westby, C. (1979). Language performance of stuttering and nonstuttering children. *Journal of Communication Disorders* 12: 133–45.

Wingate, M.E. (1964). A standard definition of stuttering. *Journal of Speech and Hearing Disorders* 29: 484–89.

Young, M. (1984). Identification of stuttering and stutterers. In R. Curlee and W. Perkins, eds., *Nature and Treatment of Stuttering; New Directions*. San Diego: College-Hill Press.

Editor's Note

The discussion section for this chapter follows Chapter 6. Because Dr. Curlee's and Dr. Ingham's papers deal with complimentary topics, a single discussion on their presentations was held at the conference.

Roger J. Ingham

6 Neuropsychology Research on Stuttering

Are There Implications for
Clinical Management?

Introduction

The purpose of this paper is to consider the contributions or implications of recent neuropsychological research on stuttering treatment. This research area also embraces the sub-area that has become known as speech-motor control research. This proves to be an unusually problematic topic because, while researchers and clinicians alike would certainly expect that this research will lead to improved treatment for stuttering, thus far it has been difficult to determine exactly how the findings can have clinical implications. The essence of the problem (at the time of writing) is that there simply do not appear to be any palpable signs that this research is yielding findings that have the potential of influencing stuttering treatment or directly changing stuttering treatment research. At the same time it is essential to add one very important qualifier: there is no inherent reason why this research area might not eventually have that effect. But, unfortunately, that future seems to be indeterminate while the dominant research orientation in neuropsychological research continues to be descriptive rather than experimental (Ventry and Schiavetti, 1986). Indeed, it is at this very basic level where a number of issues would appear to need resolutions before there is likely to be any increase in the significance of both current neuropsychological research and stuttering treatment research.

177

Only a neo-Luddite would be foolish enough to ignore the innu-
merable avenues by which research on neuropsychological processes
might benefit those who suffer from stuttering. However, there may
not be so many avenues available for detecting that benefit; at the
very least the search for reliable and effective treatments for this disorder will surely include isolating and altering whatever critical vari-
able(s) control the occurrence of this problem behavior. But it is in
the area of documenting the presence and absence of the problem
that the limited implications of current neuropsychological research
and stuttering treatment research appear to be trapped at a common
impasse. There has been a gradual recognition that treatment and
evaluation are inextricably associated and that any advances or
improvements in treatment depend on the adequacy of our therapy
evaluation methods. And it is precisely because those methods are so
wanting at the moment that stuttering treatment is at an impasse,
making it virtually impossible to fully appreciate the clinical impact
of any research domain on stuttering treatment.

Neuropsychology Research and Functional Control:
The Missing Link

One interesting feature of current speech motor and neuropsychological perspectives on stuttering is the effort that proponents of this
perspective seem to make to explain the effects of the so-called fluency-inducing procedures. These procedures are not only remark-
able because of their reliability in modifying stuttering, but because
their effects virtually characterize the disorder. More significantly,
they also subserve many current treatment systems. Efforts to
explain their effects form an important element in Starkweather's
(1987) "demands-capacities" model, are presumed to be accounted
for in Moore and Haynes's (1980) segmentation-dysfunction hypothesis, are prominent in the Neilsons' (1987) maladaptive sensory-
motor processing model, and they are critical to Kent's (1984) temporal programming disorder hypothesis. All of these proponents of

these theoretical positions certainly display concern that their hypotheses and/or models to the ameliorative effects of prolonged speech, rhythmic stimulation, masking, etc. And, of course, this is mandatory for any credible model of stuttering. Yet for some strange reason, the research that has either fostered or sustained these models has reflected surprisingly little interest in isolating the precise variables that are systematically changed by some of these powerful conditions, as well as the effect of directly manipulating and controlling these isolated variables on stuttering occurrences.

Actually, it is becoming very difficult to see where the ever-increasing number of studies that find differences between stutterers and nonstutterers with respect to their hemispheric processing, stutter-free speech, voice initiation time, and now finger tapping errors, are headed if the sources of those differences are not shown to functionally control stuttering. There are virtually no experimental studies that address this issue, let alone demonstrate, that by directly manipulating either hemispheric processing, the pauses or intervocal intervals that supposedly characterize stutterers' "fluency," voice initiation time, or heightened laryngeal activity, also will directly control the occurrence of stuttering. This is not meant to suggest that researchers should convert Kidd's (1984) findings to mean that gene splicing techniques should be used on stutterers—at least not yet. But, in principle, that is the type of research that seems to be sadly lacking and, at the very least, would make it possible to ascertain the therapy potential in this research area. More importantly, though, it would provide the field with much more information about variables that directly control stuttering—and, in turn, a method to open a window through which we might be able to peer at the less observable factors that some presume really cause this disorder.

The fact is that when physiologic and neuropsychologic differences have been found between stutterers and nonstutterers there is nothing to suggest that these differences are not merely by-products of either the presence of stuttering or experience with stuttering. For instance, much has been made of evidence that treatment results in a relative reduction in right hemisphere processing (Boberg, Yeudall,

Schopflocher and Bo-Lassen, 1983; Moore, 1984), that visual reaction measures of cerebral dominance are altered by therapy (Wilkens, Webster and Morgan, 1984), and that right hemisphere processing varies with stuttering severity (Moore, 1986). But these findings say absolutely nothing about the functional role that these changes play in stuttering or its variability. Such changes may simply be predictable epiphenomena that have no more functional importance than, say, increases in speech rate or decreases in word avoidance that might follow an effective treatment.

Even within the descriptive research framework that seems to dominate the studies discussed by Moore in Chapter 2 and Webster in Chapter 3, few attempts have been made to determine whether unusual hemispheric processing, or perhaps finger tapping errors, are unique to stutterers. Could it be that these unusual features accompany any speech-language problem and diminish when such problems are resolved? These same concerns apply to virtually all studies where such differences are found. In commenting on these studies, Rosenfield and Nudelman (1987, p. 12) made the astute observation that while there is ample evidence of *average* group differences in central and peripheral auditory function, cerebral laterality, and laryngeally-based activity (such as VOT, VIT and EMG laryngeal reaction time and cineradiographic recordings), there is virtually no evidence that any of these differences distinguish between *all* stutterers and all nonstutterers. More importantly, there seems to be growing evidence, especially among the laryngeally-oriented studies, that these average differences between adult stutterers and adult nonstutterers are not as evident among children, especially those who do not display additional speech-language problems (Ingham, 1988).

The Stuttering Measurement Crisis: Implications for Neuropsychology Research

One of the important and overlooked issues is that so much of the research in this area has relied on questionable measures of stuttering and fluency, and this is the very same reason why there is now an emerging crisis in stuttering treatment. At the source of this crisis is an issue that should impact virtually all speech physiology or neuropsychology research on stutterers: it is the continuing failure to find agreement on what is a valid and reliable measure of stuttering. This issue has dominated Perkins's publications (see Perkins, 1984; 1986) and has been greatly accentuated by Kully and Boberg's 1988 study. Together these publications have highlighted aspects of this issue which, if taken seriously, must confound many current and past endeavors to relate neurologic or physiologic variables to the appearance and nonappearance of stuttering. In Perkins's case, the issue is the validity of listener identification of stuttering, while in Kully and Boberg's case, it is the stunning lack of agreement that they found when different well-established stuttering treatment facilities made total stuttering counts on identical recordings of stutterers. As long-standing as these issues might seem (see Young, 1984), it is only now that they are causing something of a crisis in stuttering research and treatment—a crisis that desperately needs a resolution by one means or another (Ingham, 1988; 1989).

If Perkins's position is correct, then there is a major impediment to progress in most areas of treatment or nontreatment research on stuttering: since virtually all research findings have relied on listener judgments of stuttering, they must be considered suspect because there is no assurance that their data relate to valid occurrences of stuttering. If the basis of this argument is in fact correct (that is, that only stutterers can identify the sensation of "loss of control" that defines a valid stuttering event), then it may not be possible to trust the findings from the immense number of studies that have failed to check whether their subjects' stutterings were accompanied by this critical sensation.

For the moment most researchers would certainly not be willing to put aside all research findings that rely on stuttering judgments. Such a step would obviously demand supportive evidence about at least two matters: firstly, that all true stutterings *are* accompanied by "loss of control" sensations, and secondly, that it is possible to be confident that stutterers are reliable in identifying the disfluencies

that are linked to that sensation. Nevertheless, Perkins has undoubtedly raised some important issues that have even wider implications
than those he has mentioned thus far in his writings on this topic.

Meanwhile, there is certainly reason to be particularly perturbed
by the Kully and Boberg (1988) findings because if they do prove
trustworthy, then it could be that stutterings measured in one institution might not be stuttering in another institution; although that
seems to be less likely for studies whose findings have been replicated across many clinics and research centers.*

The importance of the issue raised by Kully and Boberg's study
for stuttering research and treatment, however, is almost absolutely
fundamental. To say the least, it is surely embarrassing for this discipline that there is still no standard and reliable procedure for measuring stuttering events. Since the 1940s researchers and authorities
have know that judges tend to disagree, however sophisticated they
might be, on the precise instances that they judge to be moments of
stuttering. Nonetheless, this problem has been virtually ignored
because most researchers have trusted the results of studies that
have shown that total stuttering counts can be made with satisfactory interjudge agreement. It was assumed that this meant that, at
the very least, it was possible to measure stuttering frequency with
sufficient reliability for most research and treatment studies on stuttering. However, the Kully and Boberg findings, if they are replicable, have surely torpedoed that assumption because they suggest
that different groups of clinical researchers are caught up in a form of
"folie à deux." Indeed, the magnitude of differences among stuttering counts given to some stutterers' samples from their selected clinics actually exceeds the size of changes in stuttering frequency that
many therapy studies describe as evidence of successful treatment.
Suffice to say, the continuing failure to find an agreed unit for mea-

* Since the preparation of this chapter, Ingham and Cordes (1992) have essentially
replicated Kully and Boberg's (1988) finding. The Ingham and Cordes study also
demonstrated the considerable and confounding variability in stuttering event counts
both within and across research centers.

suring stuttering limits the credibility of any research on factors that might directly influence the variability of stuttering and, thereby, identify critical variables at a more central level—if, in fact, they do exist there.

The situation in stuttering measurement is certainly not hopeless; there do exist at least some potential solutions. There are many possibilities that need to be pursued including, as this writer and colleagues have argued, the use of time interval measures of stuttering (see NINCDS, 1988). This method has been used for many years in the measurement of various types of problem behaviors where it has been difficult to achieve event-by-event interjudge agreement (Baer, Wolf and Risley, 1987). The problem with this potential solution, though, is that it may mean that it will be difficult to investigate particular stuttering events; such events would be immersed within "stuttered intervals" of speech. But that is a premature and relatively minor concern in view of the magnitude of this problem.

Meanwhile, the continuing failure to address the issue of measurement reliability has not only imperiled research involving the use of stuttering measures, but it also threatens the validity of a huge amount of research concerned with the so-called "fluent" speech or utterances of stutterers. This has been a particularly active research area because of the numerous differences that have been found between the stutter-free speech of mainly adult and adolescent stutterers and the speech of their normally fluent counterparts. However, the internal validity of many of these studies is clearly unsatisfactory. Recently, Patrick Finn and this writer (Finn and Ingham, 1989) reported a review of the procedures that most of these studies have used to select their "fluent" speech samples. Not surprisingly, it was found that virtually all of these studies have paid no attention whatsoever to the vast differences that can occur between stutter-free speech and normally fluent speech. The range of differences between these two classes of speech are, of course, well known to those of us who work in the area of stuttering treatment, but it is a difference that seems to be studiously ignored by almost all researchers investigating speech-motor variables. Even more surprising, though, was the finding that among the 93 published investigations of stutterers' stutter-free speech samples, only 54% of the reviewed studies reported on the reliability with which these samples were identified, and only 12% included checks to see whether the stutterer(s) also judged that their sample was stutter-free. If there is any research area where investigators might be expected to take into account their subjects' judgment, it is where it is essential that the speech sample in question is indeed stutter-free and perhaps normally fluent. The fact that listeners judge a sample to be stutter-free would surely be of little interest if, for instance, the subject said it contained stuttering or involved the use of an unnatural sounding speech pattern. Indeed it was interesting to find within the Finn and Ingham review only one published study (Di Simoni, 1974) in which the subject was independently judged to have spoken normally during the selected speech sample.

A particularly striking example of many of these issues occurs in a study by Caruso, Abbs and Gracco (1988). Attention is given to this study largely because its findings have received some attention in recent reviews of stuttering research (see NINCDS, 1988). The essential finding of Caruso, Abbs and Gracco's study was that when 6 stutterers and 6 nonstutterers (all males) uttered the word "sapapple," the sequence of the stutterers' upper lip, lower lip, and jaw movements differed from the consistent sequence of movements produced by their nonstutterers. Of course, it was important that this result was not confounded by stuttering, so these researchers reported that "All stutterers produced only fluent speech utterances during this test" (p. 441); yet absolutely no evidence was presented to show that these utterances *were* independently judged to be fluent, or that the stutterers also agreed that they had produced only "fluent" utterances. Consequently, as important as these findings might appear to be, they now have doubtful value because they literally hinge on an unverified claim that the stutterers' utterances were *not* contaminated by moments of stuttering. In fact, this study also failed to show that the disorderly sequence of the stutterers' movements did not resemble those that occur when the subject actually stuttered while saying "sapapple." This is not intended to be a review of Caruso, Abbs and Gracco's study, but their study actually does serve to illustrate the importance of Perkins's contention about the validity of the stutterers' judgment. That importance can be easily demonstrated by considering whether the findings from studies that failed to use stutterers' judgments would take on a different perspective if it was learned that the subject considered that the allegedly fluent sample *did* contain stuttering, and/or was not normally fluent.*

It may be the case that the uncertain reliability of stutterers' loss of control judgments will ultimately limit the use of these judgments in a treatment context, but it is just possible that stutterers' self-judgments may be quite reliable in identifying and measuring "fluency." And that could be just as important to this research area as finding a reliable and valid measure of stuttering. It should certainly be important for speech physiology or neuropsychology researchers who might be interested in learning whether stutterers are either capable or not capable of producing normally fluent speech. And in turn, that should be of considerable interest to those commentators on stuttering treatment who believe that stuttering might be incurable in some instances (Cooper, 1987).

In recent years, this writer and some colleagues have become interested in the measurement and modification of speech naturalness (Ingham and Onslow, 1985; Martin, Haroldson and Triden, 1984; Onslow and Ingham, 1987). One important premise of that research has been that normally fluent speech is likely to be speech that sounds natural to listeners *and* feels natural to the speaker. Given the validity of that premise then perhaps there are data around that offer a glimmer of hope that it might be possible to locate the essential neurologic and motoric parameters of normally fluent speech. And, of course, if that were possible then perhaps it might be possible to recognize the limits of change that can be made in a stutterer's speech. Anyhow, as a result of some studies conducted in this writer's lab (see Ingham, 1985), and more recently in

---

* It is highly significant that at least two subsequent research studies (Alfonso, 1991; McLean, Kroll and Loftus, 1990) on the kinematics of lip and jaw movement have failed to replicate the Caruso, Abbs and Gracco (1988) findings.

other laboratories (Runyan, Bell and Prosek, 1990), it is becoming clear that some listeners (not all) can make very reliable judgments of speech naturalness at repeated intervals in stutterers' speech. Furthermore, it now appears that it is possible to manipulate speech naturalness in treated stutterers so that listeners, at least, cannot recognize its difference from allegedly normally fluent speech. However, in a more recent investigation (Ingham, Ingham, Onslow and Finn, 1989) from our laboratory, we also found that three recently-treated adult stutterers could, while speaking, make repeated self-judgments of their speech naturalness with satisfactory reliability. Moreover, these subjects could produce speech that listeners and the particular stutterer judged to be highly natural sounding. But it was in the course of this study that we believe that we might have uncovered a phenomenon that could help researchers identify differences between the speech of stutterers that might *sound* normal but does not *feel* normal. The three stutterers in this study produced periods of stutter-free speech to which they gave different speech naturalness ratings. On two later and widely separated occasions, they rerated a randomized selection of recordings from these periods of speaking. It emerged that they could almost perfectly reproduce their real time speech naturalness ratings and they were more reliable than listeners in distinguishing among samples to which they originally gave different speech naturalness ratings. But that was not the only interesting finding: in the course of this study, we also had these stutterers make ratings—again, while speaking—of how naturally they *felt* that they were speaking. In essence, we wanted to see whether, when they said their stutter-free speech *sounded* highly natural, they also said that it *felt* natural. Not surprisingly, especially for those familiar with stuttering treatment, there were many occasions when subjects judged that their stutter-free speech sounded highly natural they judged that it felt quite *unnatural*. During other periods of speech, however, they judged that their natural sounding speech actually did feel quite natural. Of course, we have no way of establishing the reliability of judgments of how natural speech feels. Nonetheless, these findings suggest that highly natural sounding stutter-free speech may not always be speech that subjects judge to feel quite natural—or quite unnatural.*

Just what possible value is there in these findings for speech physiology or neuropsychology investigations of stuttering? Of course, they may have only limited value, but if this burgeoning area of research is ever going to have treatment implications, then it will certainly be necessary to know if stutterers are capable of producing speech that sounds and feels natural. That will also need to be the case if researchers are seriously interested in identifying the factors that distinguish stutter-free speech from speech that sounds normally fluent and/or natural—and, again, from speech that feels fluent and natural. These are far from trivial issues if this research area is going to search for variables that purport to induce fluency or stutter-free speech.

Therapy Variables with Implications for Neuropsychology Research

The interest that many researchers have in linking speech-motor and/or neurologic variables to the so-called fluency-inducing procedures is quite fascinating in view of the limited knowledge available about the characteristics of those procedures. This is especially true of the procedure, or set of procedures, that for the past two decades has dominated stuttering therapy for adolescents and adults. Those procedures involve the use of a speech pattern known as prolonged speech. They also include a multitude of variants of this speech pattern which Goldiamond developed in the early 1960s through the use of DAF (Goldiamond, 1965). Despite the widespread use of this procedure and its obvious—though not adequately documented—

---

* A recent study by Finn and Ingham (in press) may have provided a partial solution to this problem. They employed repeated speaking tasks using a replicable rhythmic speech pattern.

effectiveness in treating stuttering, there is virtually no information available on the precise functional variables that constitute this procedure. This is also true, incidentally, of rhythm, masking, chorus reading, and response-contingent procedures such as time out. Nevertheless, it appears that when stutterers are instructed to prolong their intervals of phonation, modify their vocal attack on consonants, and also reduce their speaking rate, then their occasions of obvious stuttering are reliably reduced. This suggests that somewhere in the midst of this (plus other speech patterns) there exists a critical variable that precisely controls the presence or absence of stuttering. And herein lies the second major crisis for stuttering therapy: the continuing failure to specify the constituents of prolonged speech so that its crucial features can be reliably identified and measured during and *after* therapy.

There are vague descriptors of the prolonged speech pattern. For example, extended voicing, soft contacts, gentle onsets, plus some acoustically and/or physiologically based systems have been developed (Agnello, 1975; 1987; Webster, 1977) for the purpose of controlling the behaviors that are supposed to fit these descriptors. However, with the exception of some very preliminary studies (Agnello, 1987; Ingham, Montgomery and Ulliana, 1983), no systematic attempts have been made to identify the necessary and sufficient components in the speech produced by these procedures, or ascertain their role in producing normal sounding stutter-free speech.

In recent years this writer and some colleagues have been trying to evaluate the effects of training stutterers and, in some cases, nonstutterers to precisely control the frequency of occurrence of phonated and nonphonated intervals of various short durations. We have found, in some instances at least, when stutterers simply increase and decrease the frequency of occurrence of these prescribed intervals, this directly increases and decreases stuttering during spontaneous speech (Ingham and Devan, 1987; Ingham, Montgomery and Ulliana, 1983). Gradually, we are learning that EGG and acoustic measures of the duration of certain components in a stutterer's speech can be very precisely controlled and self-managed. However, much of this work is also in difficulties because of increasing uncertainly about the validity of our measures of stuttering frequency.

We have certainly not been alone in attempting to identify the variables that function to control stuttering during prolonged speech or any of the other conditions (for example, Peters and Boves, 1987; Howell, El-Yaniv and Powell, 1987; Martin, Johnson, Siegel and Haroldson, 1985). It is fair to state, though, that almost all of these investigations have not sought to test whether the identified variables can be directly manipulated in the stutterer's speech and then tested to determine whether they exert functional control over stuttering. Suffice it to say that if far more concerted attempts were made to identify the precise behaviors that have functional control over stuttering (however it is measured), then perhaps researchers would be in a much better position to find the sources of control (be they at a cortical, subcortical, or whatever level) over the processes that are integral to its occurrences.

It is one thesis of this chapter that there are many areas of measurement and treatment research that should contribute to speech physiology and neuropsychology research on stuttering, rather than vice versa. One area where an interaction between both streams of research could be extremely helpful to our understanding and treatment of this disorder is untreated or, allegedly, spontaneous recovery from stuttering. There now appears to be ample justification for arguing that the so-called rate of spontaneous recovery among children who stutter is not likely to be as spontaneous or as predictable as has been believed (Ingham, 1983; Martin and Lindamood, 1986). At the very least, those persons who seem to recover spontaneously from this disorder probably do so as a result of a combination of nonenvironmental as well as environmental, or learned, factors. There are, of course, enormously important clinical implications in any evidence that might suggest that recovery is determined by nonenvironmentally- or physiologically-based variables. One of the very few studies carrying that implication is Stromsta's (1965) report from the mid 1960s which suggested that young children with disfluencies showing "lack of formant transitions and/or abnormal terminations of phonation" (1965, p. 319) were likely to be stuttering by adolescence. By contrast, those whose disfluencies did not display these features had recovered by adolescence. However, these findings are really quite inconclusive because they have never been replicated and Stromsta also failed to control for the possibility that the children who recovered also received therapy. Indeed, it is the lack of control over therapy effects, be they formal or informal, that has caused some to doubt that recovery is really spontaneous. Nevertheless, there seems to be an enormous amount that can be learned about this disorder by examining the nature of recovery among the population of so-called recovered stutterers.

One of the obvious benefits of the genetic studies is that we should be able to predict, with some measure of confidence, where and when stuttering is likely to develop. If Kidd's (1984) data are reasonably reliable—and there are some (e.g., Paul, 1988) who question that assumption—then, for instance, about 36% of male offspring of female stutterers are likely to display the disorder in childhood. Armed with this information, clinicians and researchers should be able to anticipate the emergence of stuttering and, of course, plan for its early treatment. In the second place, though, it should also be possible, retrospectively, to identify populations of recovered stutterers and gain a much better understanding of the nature of their fluent speech and the variables that distinguish them from those who failed to recover. Among the more interesting purposes in doing this research would be the possibility of gaining a better understanding of the level and quality of recovery that stutterers might achieve. Presumably, researchers could ascertain the approximate age when the subjects' recovery occurred and then test whether their speech was indeed normally fluent. For instance, it would be important to learn whether all of the acoustic, physiologic, and neuropsychologic variables that appear to characterize the adult stuttering population are also evident in the "recovered" population. If those who recover at different age levels show correlated levels of abnormality in their speech, then this might greatly influence our notions about the possibilities for recovery or, dare we say, cure. Conversely, the notion that the ultimate goal of therapy should be normally fluent speech would be greatly affected if it emerged that those who recovered in early childhood still tended to display abnormalities in their speech. It would certainly fortify the widely circulated notion (Cooper, 1987) that chronic stuttering in adults can be an essentially incurable condition, at least as far as conventional treatment procedures are concerned.

Of course, if it ultimately emerges that the principal site of dysfunction for chronic stuttering is cortically or subcortically located, then it is understandable why clinicians might favor a pharmacological approach to therapy. It is obviously premature for anyone to speculate from existing neurophysiological studies on the type of drugs that might be favored in therapy, but that has not deterred some clinicians from experimenting with various types. The recent turn towards a medical model approach to this disorder appears to be the only explanation for the sudden upsurge in "promising" drug treatment for stuttering. There are, for instance, reports that Bethanecol Chloride (Hayes, 1987) "improved fluency," and that Propanolol (Cocores, Dackis, Davies and Gold, 1986), and Carbamazepine (Goldstein, 1987) have benefitted stutterers. Yet these claims for treatment efficacy have been accompanied by absolutely no therapy evaluation data. After passing through the sad saga of haloperidol's alleged contribution to stuttering treatment (see Ingham, 1984, Ch. 11), there is a sense of déjà vu surrounding these reports. That experience should be a salutary reminder that stuttering treatment researchers have an obligation to speak out when drug treatments (or any treatments) are advocated with seemingly no regard for the complexities of stuttering therapy evaluation.

Conclusions

Despite the foregoing, there is still every reason to be confident that current research focusing on the factors influencing stutterers' abnormal speech productions and their apparent genetic susceptibility will enhance our understanding of the disorder and, ultimately, its treatment. During the interim, however, there is also reason for concern about the apparent indifference in much of this research towards notions of internal and external validity. Topping the list of these concerns is the problem of reliably identifying and measuring stuttering. When that almost fundamental issue is resolved, then there still remains an enormous amount to learn about the so-called fluency-inducing conditions; if only to identify the variables that directly manipulate stuttering and, thereby, monitor the effect of that manipulation on the systems that subserve speech production—whatever the level. That process alone would benefit stuttering treatment enormously.

There is little doubt that stuttering treatment needs an infusion of new ideas. A strong case can be made to support the claim that understanding the function and effects of stuttering treatment is no better than it was 10 or 15 years ago. In fact, it might be going backwards if the number of published reports on stuttering therapy is an indicator. In the past 5 years, for instance, there has been a 50% decline in the number of such reports when compared with two previous 5-year periods (Ingham, 1988). There are many reasons for this, but at the forefront is our discipline's failure to develop clinically valid measures of speech performance, the continuing failure to operationalize and systematically investigate our treatment agents, and the apparent indifference to the complex issues associated with identifying the long-term effects of treatment. The failure to address these issues may have not only damaged the development of clinically effective treatments, but also the quality of stuttering treatment. Part of the reason why the zeitgeist in stuttering research has shifted to the speech-motor and/or neuropsychology areas may well be because many have perceived that behaviorally-based stuttering treatments have been, at best, only partially effective. That may well be a perfectly predictable result of our partial approach to treatment research.

In concluding this chapter it may be useful to raise one other concern about stuttering therapy, especially because it relates to issues that have surfaced in discussions about other chapters in this book. It seems that very gradually our field has developed a prescription-driven approach to therapy evaluation. Wittingly or unwittingly, we have begun to prescribe the goals of therapy as stutter-free and relatively normal sounding speech that is durable across speaking situations and over a time span that seems to run from six months to two years. Perhaps our orientation to therapy and even the nature of the problem might change considerably if therapy was, as Don Baer (1988; 1989) has recently suggested, complaint driven. The basis of Baer's notion is that therapy is usually only applied to those individuals for whom the disorder has become so problematic that treatment is needed to stop them from complaining (to therapists or others) about it. Could it be, therefore, that the direction for treatment should come from the source of the complaint and that the goals of therapy should be the extent to which the stutterer ceases to be aggravated by those sources? We have shaped a great deal of our therapy towards the objective of normally fluent speech—which certainly *seems* to be a credible objective. But it is just possible that the achievement of normally fluent speech is not the concern of the person who seeks treatment. Indeed, it may well be the case that treatment achieves its purpose when persons who stutter simply find it possible to do those tasks that had previously caused them to complain about their speech.

It might also be the case that when stutterers are concerned about the sensation of loss of control, they are not complaining about stuttering as such, but about the sensation of loss of control. Equally, it may be that when other stutterers complain about their speech, they are not the least bit concerned about the sensation of loss of control, but about the reaction that it causes in others. The obvious danger in this type of speculation is that it may lead to the problems that befell stuttering treatment when it was dictated by those who insisted that stuttering is a problem for the listener, not the speaker. However, there is also ample reason to be concerned that researchers do not lose touch with the notion of a "problem behavior" when we address the issue of treatment.

That problem behavior may take different forms at different times in treatment. For instance, it often seems to be the case that the point at which that problem disappears for many treated stutterers is not when stutter-free and even normal sounding speech is achieved, but when the cost or effort involved in maintaining their improved speech is reduced. Putting aside the measurement issues that were mentioned earlier, it does seem that the point of interest in stuttering treatment is gradually starting to shift towards a concern about the stutterer's sensation of control during speech. But it is not so much the sensation of loss of control as the sensation of excessive control; that is, the control that treated stutterers need to exert over their speech in order to sustain the fluency gained by some treatments. Somehow or other treatment researchers need to be able to identify the characteristics of this excessive control and distinguish it from the characteristics of normal control. Just when and how these distinguishing characteristics can be located and then related to treatment might turn out to be the major contribution that neuropsychology research can make to stuttering therapy.

References

Agnello, J.G. (1975). Voice onset and voice termination features of stutterers. In L.M. Webster (ed.), *Proceedings of the Hayes Martin Conference on Vocal Tract Dynamics in Stuttering*. New York: Speech and Hearing Institute.

———. (1987). A comprehensive computer program for facilitating fluency in stutterers. In H.F.M. Peters and W. Hulstijn (eds.), *Speech Motor Dynamics in Stuttering* (pp. 307–15). New York: Springer-Verlag.

Alfonso, P.J. (1991). Implications of the concepts underlying task-dynamic modeling on kinematic studies of stuttering. In H.F.M. Peters, W. Hulstijn and C.W. Starkweather (eds.), *Speech Motor Control and Stuttering* (pp. 307–15). Amsterdam: Springer-Verlag.

Baer, D.M. (1988). If you know why you're changing a behavior, you'll know when you've changed it enough. *Behavioral Assessment* 10: 219–23.

———. (1989). The critical issue in treatment efficacy is knowing why treatment was applied: a student's response to Roger Ingham. Paper read to American Speech-Language-Hearing Foundation Conference on Treatment Efficacy, San Antonio, Texas, March 17.

Baer, D.M., Wolf, M.M. and Risley, T.R. (1987). Some still-current dimensions of applied behavior analysis. *Journal of Applied Behavior Analysis* 20: 313–27.

Boberg, E., Yeudall, L.T., Schopflocher, D. and Bo-Lassen, P. (1983). The effect of an intensive behavioral program on the distribution of EEG alpha power in stutterers during the processing of verbal and visuospatial information. *Journal of Fluency Disorders* 8: 245–63.

Caruso, A.J., Abbs, J.H. and Gracco, V.L. (1988). Kinematic analysis of multiple movement coordination during speech in stutterers. *Brain* 111: 439–55

Cocores, J.A., Dackis, C.A., Davies, R. and Gold, M.S. (1986). Propranolol and stuttering. *American Journal of Psychiatry* 143: 1071–72.

Cooper, E.B. (1987). The Chronic Perseverative Stuttering Syndrome; incurable stuttering. *Journal of Fluency Disorders* 12: 381–88.

Di Simoni, F.G. (1974). Preliminary study of certain timing relationships in the speech of stutterers. *Journal of Acoustical Society of America* 56: 695–96.

Finn, P., and Ingham, R.J. (1989). The selection of "fluent" samples in research on stuttering: conceptual and methodological considerations. *Journal of Speech and Hearing Research* 32: 401–18.

———. (in press). Stutterers' self-ratings of how natural speech sounds and feels. *Journal of Speech and Hearing Research.*

Goldiamond, I. (1965). Stuttering and fluency as manipulatable operant response classes. In L. Krasner and L.P. Ullmann (eds.), *Research in Behavior Modification* (pp. 106–56), New York: Holt, Rinehart and Winston.

Goldstein, J.A. (1987). Carbamazepine treatment for stuttering. *Journal of Clinical Psychiatry* 48: 39

Hayes, P. (1987). Bethanecol chloride in treatment of stuttering. *The Lancet*, p. 271, January 31.

Howell, P., El-Yaniv, N. and Powell, D.J. (1987). Factors affecting fluency in stutterers when speaking under altered auditory feedback. In H.F.M. Peters and W. Hulstijn (eds.), *Speech Motors Dynamics in Stuttering* (pp. 361–69). New York: Springer-Verlag.

Ingham, R.J. (1983). Spontaneous remission of stuttering: When will the Emperor realize he has no clothes on? In D. Prins and R.J. Ingham (eds.), *Treatment of Stuttering in Early Childhood: Methods and Issues* (pp. 113–40) San Diego: College-Hill Press.

———. (1984). *Stuttering and Behavior Therapy: Current Status and Experimental Foundations.* San Diego: College-Hill Press.

———. (1985). Stuttering treatment outcome evaluation: closing the credibility gap. *Seminars in Speech and Language* 6: 105–23.

———. (1988). Research on stuttering treatment for adults and adolescents:

A perspective on how to overcome a malaise. Paper read to NINCDS workshop "Research needs in stuttering: roadblocks and future directions." Bethesda, Maryland, September 15.

———. (1989). Theoretical, methodological, and ethical issues in treatment efficacy research: stuttering therapy as a case study. Keynote address to American Speech-Language-Hearing Foundation Conference on Treatment Efficacy. San Antonio, Texas, March 17.

Ingham, R.J. and Cordes, A.K. (1992). Interclinic differences in stuttering-events counts. *Journal of Fluency Disorders* 17: 171–76.

Ingham, R.J. and Devan, D. (1987). Phonated and nonphonated interval modifications in the speech of stutterers. Paper read to the American Speech-Language-Hearing Association Annual Convention, New Orleans, November 22.

Ingham, R.J., Ingham, J.C., Onslow, M. and Finn, P. (1989). Stutterers' self-ratings of speech naturalness: assessing effects and reliability. *Journal of Speech and Hearing Research* 32: 419–31.

Ingham, R.J., Montgomery, J. and Ulliana, L. (1983). The effect of manipulating phonation duration on stuttering. *Journal of Speech and Hearing Research* 26: 579–587.

Ingham, R.J. and Onslow, M. (1985). Measurement and modification of speech naturalness during stuttering therapy. *Journal of Speech and Hearing Disorders* 50: 261–81.

Kent, R.D. (1984). Stuttering as a temporal programming disorder. In R.F. Curlee and W.H. Perkins (eds.), *Nature and Treatment of Stuttering: New Directions* (pp. 283–301) San Diego: College-Hill Press.

Kidd, K.K. (1984). Stuttering as a genetic disorder. In R.F. Curlee and W.H. Perkins (eds.), *Nature and Treatment of Stuttering: New Directions* (pp. 149–69). San Diego: College-Hill Press.

Kully, D. and Boberg, E. (1988). An investigation of interclinic agreement in the identification of fluent and stuttered syllables. *Journal of Fluency Disorders* 13: 309–18.

Martin, R.R., Haroldson, S.K. and Triden, K.A. (1984). Stuttering and speech naturalness. *Journal of Speech and Hearing Disorders* 49: 53–58.

Martin, R.R., Johnson, L.J., Siegel, G.M. and Haroldson, S.K. (1985). Auditory stimulation, rhythm, and stuttering. *Journal of Speech and Hearing Research* 28: 487–95.

Martin, R.R. and Lindamood, L.P. (1986). Stuttering and spontaneous recovery: implications for the Speech-Language Pathologist. *Language, Speech, and Hearing Services in Schools* 17: 207–18.

McLean, M.D., Kroll, R.M. and Loftus, N.S. (1990) Kinematic analysis of lip closure in stutterers' fluent speech. *Journal of Speech and Hearing Research* 33: 755–60.

Moore, W.H., Jr. (1984). Hemispheric alpha asymmetries during an electromyographic biofeedback procedure for stuttering. *Journal of Fluency Disorders* 17: 143–62.

————. (1986). Hemispheric alpha asymmetries of stutterers and non-stutterers for the recall and recognition of words and connected reading passages: Some relationships to severity of stuttering. *Journal of Fluency Disorders* 11: 71–89.

Moore, W.H., Jr. and Haynes, W.C. (1980). Alpha hemispheric asymmetry and stuttering: some support from a segmentation dysfunction hypothesis. *Journal of Speech and Hearing Research* 23: 229–247.

Neilson, M.D. and Neilson, P.D. (1987). Speech motor control and stuttering: a computational model of adaptive sensory-motor processing. *Speech Communication* 6: 325–333.

NINCDS. (1988). Research needs in stuttering: roadblocks and future directions. Workshop sponsored by National Institute of Neurological and Communicative Disorders and Stroke, Bethesda, Maryland, September 14–15.

Onslow, M. and Ingham, R.J. (1987). Speech quality measurement and the management of stuttering. *Journal of Speech and Hearing Disorders* 51: 2–17.

Pauls, D.L. (1988). A review of the evidence for genetic factors in stuttering. Paper read to NINCDS workshop, "Research needs in stuttering: roadblocks and future directions." Bethesda, Maryland, September 14–15.

Perkins, W.H. (1984). Stuttering as a categorical event: barking up the wrong tree—reply to Wingate. *Journal of Speech and Hearing Disorders* 49: 431–34.

————. (1986). More bite for a bark: Epilogue to Martin and Haroldson's Letter. *Journal of Speech and Hearing Disorders* 51: 190–91.

Peters, H.F.M. and Boves, L. (1987). Aerodynamic functions in fluent speech utterances of stutterers and nonstutterers in different speech conditions. In H.F.M. Peters and W. Hulstijn (eds.), *Speech Motor Dynamics in Stuttering* (pp. 229–244). New York: Springer-Verlag.

Rosenfield, D.B., and Nudelman, H.B. (1987). Neuropsychological models of speech dysfluency. In L. Rustin, H. Purser, and D. Rowley (eds.), *Progress in the Treatment of Fluency Disorders* (pp. 3–18). London: Taylor and Francis.

Runyan, C.M., Bell, J.N. and Prosek, R.A. (1990). Speech naturalness ratings of treated stutterers. *Journal of Speech and Hearing Disorders* 55: 434–38.

Starkweather, C.W. (1987). *Fluency and Stuttering*. Englewood Cliffs, New Jersey: Prentice Hall.

Stromsta, C. (1965). A spectrographic study of dysfluencies labeled as stuttering by parents. *De Therapia Vocis et Loquelae* (Proceedings XIII International Congress of Logopedics and Phoniatrics, Vienna), Vol. 1, 317–19.

Ventry, I.M. and Schiavetti, N. (1986). *Evaluating Research in Speech Pathology and Audiology*, 2nd. ed. New York: Macmillan.

Webster, R.L. (1977). A few observations on the manipulation of speech response characteristics in stutterers. *Journal of Communication Disorders* 10: 73–78.

Wilkens, C., Webster, R.L. and Morgan, B.T. (1984). Cerebral lateralization of visual stimulus recognition in stutterers and fluent speakers. *Journal of Fluency Disorders* 9: 131–41.

Young, M.A. (1984). Identification of stuttering and stutterers. In R.F. Curlee and W.H. Perkins (eds.), *Nature and Treatment of Stuttering: New Directions* (pp. 13–30). San Diego: College-Hill Press.

Discussion

R. Kroll: The original titles of the talks were "Implications for Assessment" and "Implications for Clinical Management." Most of the group members were in agreement that you in fact did not address clinical implications but rather provided us with a rather lengthy treatise on current applications to therapy and to diagnosis. We would like to know why you chose to deal with the topic in that way?

R. Curlee: I do not think that I was as clear as Roger in saying that my opinion is that the clinical implications of the information that we have received at this meeting are unknown. Period!

R. Ingham: I had great difficulty in dealing with some of the issues emerging in this area because I genuinely looked for clinical implications. I am certainly willing to be persuaded that there are implications. And I certainly agree that there are individuals who believe that there are strong clinical implications among the findings. I want to say again though, that at the moment I am yet to be persuaded, by the evidence that I have seen, that those implications are strong enough to affect what I see to be the current issues in stuttering treatment, or indeed have an impact on stuttering treatment. The point that I wanted to make is that the whole area of stuttering is hamstrung, absolutely, by the failure to come to terms with the issue of

measuring stuttering. This issue spills into all areas of stuttering research, of treatment. If we do not know the reliability
with which we can measure those dependent variables, and
those dependent variables are the critical variables in therapy
then I have some difficulty at the moment in getting beyond
this issue in evaluating research in this area. I think that is my
concern.

R. Kroll: Roger and Dick [Curlee], as you probably know better than I
do, we have a lot of schisms in speech pathology, especially in
the area of stuttering research, theory and therapy. Are we
tonight witnessing an historic occasion, the inauguration of a
new schism or rift between the Behaviorists and the Neuro-
physiologists, where one rejects the others' work out of hand
and where we divide ourselves into various camps? As an
addendum to that question, given the limitations of the current
procedures and research in electrophysiology, as you have
pointed out, can you dig deep, deep down, and tell us if you see
anything positive coming out of that work?

R. Ingham: I am sure that I can find the place in my paper, where I
said that I am extremely hopeful that this area will provide
those critical variables that are relevant to treatment. I am certain that they are not going to be those that we currently use in
treatment. I am absolutely positive of that. I think that I anticipate most the marrying of the developments that are taking
place in neuropsychology research and in treatment. I certainly
do not want to foster a schism. If there was an implication
about behavioral based treatments versus some sort of physiological treatment then that is an archaic notion. The separating
of behavior, physiology and functional physiology is not a
notion I subscribe to at all. I rather feel that we do have some
clues in the current treatment procedures that should be pursued. We need to see whether the variables that seem to function in that context can give us an inroad, or help us to look at

what is transpiring at the neurophysiological level. I am totally uncommitted to either position about that.

R. Curlee: I feel, like Roger, that I was unsuccessful in expressing my personal interest and appreciation for much of the physiological and neuropsychological research that is going forward. I think it has real promise for helping us better understand the nature of stuttering. In terms of clinical diagnosis, I also tried to make clear in my presentation, and perhaps failed, that I think it is essential that we use empirical bases for deciding how we treat clients. My own reading of the literature is that much of the clinical work that has gone on, particularly prior to 1960, was theory driven. It was based on people's presumption of the nature of stuttering and people were directing their treatment approaches and diagnostic approaches to those assumptions or presumptions about the nature of stuttering.

At this time, many of us feel that those ideas about the nature of stuttering are not very useful. In my judgment we should not try to pattern our clinical work after our beliefs about the nature of stuttering. I think that it is much more important to continue to do what is effective clinically, and I think our diagnostic assessments need to have some clinically relevant purpose. Why would I assess someone? I want to assess someone to identify whether or not the person stutters, determine the severity of the problem and perhaps identify the scope of the problem. Is it possible to identify issues or factors in the environment that might be exacerbating or maintaining the problem and try to change some of those? Other than these, I know of no other reasons to do a clinical assessment. As far as I am concerned, there is no evidence, that I have heard or that I have read, which shows that the physiological or the neuropsychological measures that we have been talking about are related to clinical assessment of stutterers or if any are even causally related to stuttering. And while I am excited about potential breakthroughs from such information, I still believe

that it is premature to change our diagnostic procedures, particularly with young children, particularly with incipient stutterers, on the basis of data that have been primarily obtained from
adults.

W. Moore: Why did you accept the job to discuss the implications of
this research if you had a predetermined bias that there were no
implications? That was your job and you did not do it, as it was
Roger's.

R. Curlee: I accept your opinion Skip.

W. Moore: I do not accept yours.

Question from floor to W. Moore: Why didn't you or somebody else
help him?

W. Moore: That was his job. He accepted it. I gave you some dis-
claimers before I got into my presentation.

R. Ingham: I thought I gave a pretty strong disclaimer when I stood
up. I have spent a considerable amount of time reading the
research. I pride myself on trying to keep abreast of most of it
and trying to see its clinical implications. I think that the major
issues that face us at the moment are to be able to precisely
identify what is transpiring in stuttering behavior. Being able to
measure stuttering reliably is a starting point.

W. Moore: That is a different issue.

R. Ingham: No, it is not a different issue. It is critical because it is the
very basis for assessing effects of therapy or measuring any clinical implications from the work discussed here. At the moment,
we are absolutely stymied. Failure to resolve this issue also
directly affects the research that is being done in numerous

research laboratories. I am really uncomfortable about accepting the data from the Edmonton crew (Kully and Boberg, 1988), but if I accept this as evidence, then we are simply not talking to each other: different laboratories are referring to different events when they research stuttering. I think that is a fundamental issue. You were at the (NIH) conference in Washington when we looked at the roadblocks to research; this issue just came up, over and over again. I do not know what else to say at this point. When we have come to terms with that issue, and gotten beyond that issue, then we are going to be in a much better position to be able to evaluate the clinical implications.

W. *Moore:* You have to deal with this research. Have you read it? There are lots of studies. There are not just three or four or five. There are many. Have you looked at how stuttering was measured in all those investigations? Have you related that to the procedures? Have you offered a better procedure? I wonder?

R. *Ingham:* For measuring stuttering?

W. *Moore:* How much time have you spent in an electrophysiological laboratory gathering data or developing a better procedure?

R. *Ingham:* Surely nobody would suggest that people have to be in the same type of laboratories to evaluate research.

W. *Moore:* Science needs better procedures, not unsubstantiated criticism from folks that don't address the issue. You know that.

R. *Ingham:* Everybody has a right to their opinion when interpreting the data. The data are there to be interpreted. The methodologies are there to look at. Everybody has a right to be able to comment on the methodologies. Nobody would dispute that this area of work might not ultimately have clinical value. I am not disputing that. Can I say that again? I am not disputing that this area of work might not have clinical value. Okay? I do not have any difficulty in accepting that it might have clinical value in the future.

W. Moore: Some of us wish that you had addressed the issues that were advertised here.

R. Curlee: Let me interrupt and say that my comment about a "lazy left hemisphere" was intended to be a funny, flippant remark. If I offended you, I apologize. I respect your work, but in my opinion, your work is not ready for clinical application at this time. That is my opinion.

W. Moore: Was the word that you used, clinical application or clinical implication? Does the conference brochure say *application* or *implication*? I thought it said *implication*.

R. Curlee: It says implication, I believe.

H. Gregory: I have a question that I hope will lead us to think about the future. It is addressed to you both. Do you think that the demands capacity model might be a good model, looking to the future, that will afford a working relationship between researchers and clinicians in neuropsychology, cognitive psychology and speech-language pathology?

R. Curlee: I can answer that very briefly. My own feeling is that this is a most useful and productive kind of framework or model framework that, at least to me, seems to make sense at this time. I am not sure how successful or useful this model is going to be in the future because I do not think you can predict scientific advances. One of the things that gives me reason to believe in this model's utility is that so many different people, looking at stuttering from a wide range of different perspectives, are using the same kinds of ideas to model the differences that we observe in stuttered and nonstuttered speech, and between stutterers and nonstutterers. My personal view is that this is a very useful model and that it will likely continue to be very useful in the future.

R. Ingham: I really think it does have applications in a number of ways. It is certainly fostering a lot of interest at the moment.

H. Gregory: I would like to address my next question to Dr. Ingham. If through research we could come close to measuring the kinds of variables, speech and otherwise, in the way you would like, if we could do that at the beginning of therapy, during therapy and after therapy, if we could also make neuropsychological measurements during that period, if we could describe very carefully the process of therapy, why we think some cases did not respond well, how that relates to the data that we have and so forth, do you think that this sounds like a fruitful approach to research in the future?

R. Ingham: Yes, that is the sort of multi-level measurement system that I really do think offers exciting possibilities, particularly if it were possible to gain measures at all levels—cortical, sub-cortical, and throughout the motor system—concurrent with behavior. There are serious problems associated with that and I think that the people working at the level of EEG work are very aware of this. Gaining real time access to precisely what is transpiring during speech, presents some mountainous problems at the moment. But, in principle, I believe that is exactly the sort of way in which we will learn what goes on. I do not see, for some time, our being able to get over the problem of observer judgments or speaker judgments, one of the principal dependent variables. I know that presents serious problems. How do we get around that? The dream is that there will be physiological markers and/or neurologic markers for each occasion of stuttering. If that materialized, that would be one of the most massive breakthroughs, at the clinical and theoretical level, for the whole disorder. That may come about through multi-level measuring of the type that you were talking about.

_____

A. Caruso: Roger, one of the arguments that you make, a valid point that I agree with, is the difficulties in accurately measuring both stuttered and fluent behavior. At the same time you seem to be criticizing one small part of the research we did, albeit a critical portion, because there were no accurate or reliable measures of fluent behavior. We anxiously await your contributions to the further development of those areas so that we can use them in our work. We used what was available at the time, but we continue to want to refine it in the future, as I hope you will want to continue to refine some of your behavioral observations, given the underlying neuropsychology and the underlying motor control.

Now, I will ask a question. Do you think it would be a reasonable treatment approach to look at the treatment strategies or the treatments themselves that are affected in the stuttering therapy and then relate physiological factors to them? In essence, the stuttering treatment factors would act as independent variables.

R. Ingham: Precisely! Absolutely! Let me say that the reason I chose to talk about your paper was because I admired the paper immensely. Let me tell you a little story about it. I first came across it as a reviewer for ASHA convention papers. The last paper that I can recall that was as creative as yours, was a paper by Chuck Reed—a paper that I remember vividly. Anyhow I am certain your study can be replicated without that problem. The problem, it seems to me, is one that characterizes many papers; it is overlooking the simple act of verification (which I'm certain you appreciate is one of the fundamental factors in methodology); just verifying that the behaviors you measured *were* the behaviors. I really think that the linkage between that sort of methodology and the procedures, that we can hopefully drag out of the therapy process, is the sort of thing that can lead us towards finding the very precise controls that exist. My criticisms, contrary to what might have come across here, are really directed toward stuttering treatment as much as towards any other area because I think stuttering treatment is in a damn mess. We have failed to identify and quantify the precise characteristics that we are supposed to be controlling and modifying in therapy. Frankly, I do not know how on earth people know what they are doing in therapy. There are no data available describing how reliable people are in identifying gentle onsets, or judging soft contacts and so forth. So, in order for some of us to be able to talk to you, we really have to get our own house in order. I think there are some areas you can contribute to us, but we have to have our house in order before we can receive them.

A. Caruso: Thank you Roger. I should tell you, because I promised the group I would say this, that the reaction of the group to both presentations was split. I think that perhaps a slight majority of the group were somewhat discouraged in what they perceived to be the tenor of your comments. A somewhat lesser portion of the group was encouraged by some of the things both of you said.

A. Kroll: I would just like to add a small comment to that, Tony, because in my group some members were depressed almost to the point of pre-hospital admission. I am not trying to fool here. I think that what the summation of the conference seems to be saying to us as researchers and clinicians is that we do not know what we are measuring, we do not know how to assess, we do not know how to measure our treatment effects, and we question the link between the neurophysiological research and the treatment research. It was at times a discouraging and depressing kind of conversation.

A. Caruso: One of the concerns was a perception, on the part of many of the people in the group, that you were advocating an isolated, single, exclusive track for research versus room for many different approaches. Would you agree that there are other types of research which continue to be important and should be maintained?

R. Curlee: I do not think anyone knows what approach or what questions are going to yield the most fruitful kinds of insight into the nature of stuttering or its treatment. So, I have always believed that we should make sure that we keep as many different methods of study of stuttering going as is fiscally possible. Let me also comment that I do not think there is any doubt that there is a relationship between physiological events and behavioral events. I believe this as an assumption, but I do not think we know what the functional relationships between those events are, right now. It is not a question of whether or not there is a relationship. It is a question, in my judgment, that we do not know what they are.

H. Gregory: Do either one of you have any recommendations on how to find the neuropsychological variables underlying some of the fluency enhancing procedures? Can you think of other ways to make meaning of the kinds of research that is being reported here, ways that will enable us to really understand the implications for and applications to evaluation and treatment?

R. Curlee: Let me add something, Hugo. I think that one of the most important things that needs to be done, with neuropsychological and physiological research is to start looking at young children, who are just beginning to stutter. This is the age group with which we have most of our clinical success. This is also the age group about which we know very little. It would be incredibly useful if we were able to find some physiological or neuropsychological signatures that distinguish between those children who are going to remit without, or with minimal professional intervention, and those who are not going to remit without such intervention. This will require longitudinal studies. The better able we are to manage such problems in young children effectively and efficiently, the better off people who stutter are going to be.

R. Ingham: Just to reiterate what was also in my paper, and it follows from what Dick just said. I think that there is such a tremendous amount to be learned by looking at those people that have recovered from the disorder and getting a much better understanding of just what has transpired; what is transpiring in their speech and in their entire system of speech production. That should tell us a lot more than it has thus far. There should be a huge pool of these people.

A. Caruso: Some of those people you need for that study may be inaccessible. It would seem to me, based on my clinical experience, that the vast majority of children who begin stuttering and spontaneously recover from stuttering, do so without interaction with the speech clinician. Therefore, even those children who do come into the speech clinic and do recover, either spontaneously or otherwise, may represent a restricted sub-group that is similar to the adults, but at a different level. It is a methodological problem. I agree that those children need to be looked at, but perhaps we would be better served if we looked at normal children who are developing fluency in longitudinal studies. We could gather 12–13 months of data.

R. Ingham: That is exactly the kind of work that I think should be done. As I alluded to in my paper, we now have pretty good genetic information. Genetic studies, if we use them, should be able to give us strong indicators as to where and when we can expect the occurrence of stuttering. We should be in a position to marshall our forces or our monitoring systems, to be able to watch that group. I think that is the great possibility in all of that work.

Questions from the Floor

A. Rochet: Drs. Curlee and Ingham, this is just a comment, not a question. I am Anne Putnam Rochet from the University of Alberta. This goes back to one of Dr. Kroll's initial questions; the idea of implication, and the semantic distinctions made here. It seems to me that the flip-side of implication is inference, and inference is a very dangerous thing on which to apply anything. I thank you very much for your critical comments tonight. I appreciate the opportunity to have heard them and I appreciate the courage that it took to say them.

L. Lavallee: Thank you very much for your paper. My name is Larry Lavallee. I wonder how you would view the conclusion that I am getting from the papers presented; that there is a broad spectrum type problem of stuttering. How would you change the definition of what we call stuttering? Might you define the problem as a communication problem with speech being one variable and affecting other processes?

R. Curlee: Personally, as a clinician, I see stuttering as a communication problem. I have believed for a long time that Joe Sheehan's 1958 description of stuttering as a combination of three different types of symptoms, one of which involves speech disruption, one of which involves emotional reactions to those speech disruptions and to speaking situations, and thirdly, the kinds of self-concepts or beliefs about oneself that one develops as a result of growing up with these kinds of speech disruptions, is a useful clinical concept. I am not sure what you mean by "stuttering as a broad spectrum disorder."

L. Lavallee: I was indicating that it might affect other physiological processes. For example, it is often referred to as secondary behavior, yet we have not defined stuttering as involving secondary behaviors. There is no proof of any secondary behaviors.

R. Curlee: In my paper I frequently used the words "stutterer's problem," or "the stuttering problem." I tried to imply that the problem of stuttering frequently extends beyond the disruptions in speech that we observe. For example, in support of Don Baer's idea, we need to keep a problem-oriented approach in our clinical management of stutterers. This does not mean that we would not try to help them with their speech. We need to find out what it is about their speech, what it is about their attempts to communicate, to express themselves, that is bothering them, and then figure out how we can assist them, regardless of what particular techniques we choose to use.

H. Goldberg: I am Herb Goldberg from the Foundation for Fluency. I am really interested in one facet of your presentation about being able to measure stuttering by the feelings of the client, instead of fluency counting by the speech pathologist. The important thing is not complete fluency but to reach a comfort level that the client is satisfied with. The question I want to ask is what percentage of speech pathologists do you feel agree with this way of dealing with stuttering?

R. Ingham: I think that in many ways the people working in recently developed approaches to stuttering treatment have received— and perhaps deservedly—something of a bad rap for being single-minded in their measurement approaches. I think what has been missed by many is that we have been constantly listening to what has been "going on" with our data; or what has been going on with clients in treatment. We have been constantly trying to find ways to quantify the sorts of things that clients seem concerned with; trying to see whether we can get those concerns into a form so that we can do something about them; not in a form where they are amorphous concepts that can't be operationalized, so that we can't do anything about them.

I know that some people, including myself, and others working with me, have been aware for a long time of the problems
associated with stuttering treatment. We have been at the brunt
of quite a good deal of criticism about it. We have been trying
to respond to that, trying to come to terms with some of these
issues and trying to see whether they are pertinent variables or
not, by putting them into laboratories wherever we can. One of
the points that has been missed about the developments that
took place in that era—and I do not want to shift the focus of
this conference—is that there has been colossal skepticism on
the part of the people who have been developing and assessing
the procedures in this area. They have been just as bothered,
even more bothered in many instances, by what has transpired,
what cannot be done, and the limitations associated with what
is being done. The tragedy is that that has not been conveyed in
clinical reports.

C. Mateer: I have a comment. I am not sure it is a question but I
would be interested in your response. I feel I have done some
basic science research and a lot of applied clinical research
lately, not in the area of stuttering but in cognitive treatments,
attention and memory functions. I certainly appreciate the difficulty in bridging the gap between the basic science of what are
attentional mechanisms and how we can treat them. I guess
what I am hearing from you, and I will call you clinicians
because that is how I am seeing you although I realize you are
clinical researchers, are statements like, "show me that this is
relative" or "prove to me that this is relevant" or "tell me how I
can use this." What I would hope for is more statements of
commitment, communication and cooperation. It is time to set
up some cooperative studies whereby you take some parameter
coming out of physiology or out of the motor control work and
say, "let's apply that in a clinical setting." I really believe that
therapeutic studies and clinical studies are not going to come
out of laboratories. They will have to come out of the clinic. I

am concerned to hear the amount of strife and discomfort between people who are doing the more "basic" science versus the more "applied" clinical science.

R. Ingham: I can only speak for the sort of area we are working in. Our research lab is literally linked with our clinic. I think that in the stream of research that I have been associated with in Australia and here, there has been this constant to-ing and fro-ing between the clinic and the laboratory. I think that has been enormously productive for our stuttering treatment work. In the midst of all this, we really have developed some fairly effective approaches to the control of this problem behavior primarily as a result of a lot of clinical research. I mean it is not all disaster. The treatment/research area, at the moment though, is in a rather disastrous state because it has not come to terms with some of the issues I mentioned. There is a fertile and constant association going on between research and clinical activity in many places that I am familiar with. Certainly, that is true in Edmonton.

L. Gibson: One of the things that I have felt that a lot of the people here have been hoping to get, was some way of being able to go back Monday morning with something a little bit different, to be able to try and deal with their clients. One of the things I would like to offer is that for me, as a stutterer, who grew up feeling an absolute failure because I was told it was my behavior, that there was no "it" and if I did not do "it" I would not stutter. I find it very hopeful, and helpful to be told that there is work being done in the neuropsychological field.

Someday I would like to look upon this as a disorder, something that does indeed happen to me and that there is an "it" like cancer or dyslexia or arthritis. Now, we have a lot of behaviors that accompany that; let's get down to work on it. There are some stutterers who do not like being told it is physiological because for them it is like being told they can do nothing about it. From this research, at least, it sounds like there is hope in the future. Maybe we can even do something about the physiological aspect. In the meantime, we need to work on the stuttering behavior. What we can remove, at least from some stutterers, is a tremendous burden of guilt and failure and I find that hopeful. Thank you.

William H. Perkins

7   What Is Stuttering and Why?

For half a century, we have proceeded on the premise that clinicians can detect stuttering as well, if not better, than stutterers. In fact, we are so confident that we know what stuttering is that we train stutterers to agree with us as to whether or not they have stuttered. Could it be that our premise is wrong? Can we only guess whether or not we have heard stuttering? Is it only the stutterer who knows for sure and then only when it happens? And is it involuntary disruption that tells the stutterer whether he has really stuttered or just sounds as if he has? If this is true, it leads to the premise that stuttering is not determined by quantity of syllable disfluency but by quality. Why is stuttered speech categorically different from nonstuttered speech? Is it a qualitative, not a quantitative difference?

To begin, we need to explain all of the phenomena of stuttering, not just selected samples and to take seriously our clinical knowledge as well as our experimental knowledge. This has rarely been done before. For example, how many studies have attempted to account for how stuttered and nonstuttered speech are different, even when they sound alike as they do when stutterers fake their stuttering and can tell the difference? Why do stutterers have "good days" and "bad days?" Why does time pressure play such a pivotal role in at least chronic stuttering? Why does the topography of stuttering vary, sometimes within the same individual on the same utterance? What terminates as well as initiates an occurrence? Why do peak periods of onset of stuttering parallel language acquisition so closely? Why is remittance of stuttering all but over by the end of language acquisition? Why, subsequent to language acquisition, does stuttering become chronic? Beyond these constraints our knowledge of stuttering phenomena imposes on possible explanations are also the constraints imposed from related fields of study: psycholinguistics, cognitive science, neuroscience, genetics, evolutionary science, for instance. Given these constraints, the possible answers are severely restricted.

To explain these aspects of stuttering requires explaining how the flow of speech is processed in the brain. I find much of the cutting edge research immensely impressive. My problem is that I just do not know how to make sense of it. I wonder how we are going to recognize an important difference in brain function when we find it, if we do not know the brain functions that have to be performed when speech is fluent, or normally disfluent, or is stuttered, or just sounds like it is stuttered? Since I have no certainty which parts of the brain perform which speech-flow function, what I propose to do is start with the functions the brain must necessarily perform to meet the constraints laid down. The brain operates in modules, so the modules relevant to disruptions of speech flow need to be delineated. Starting with the obvious, speech is obviously the oral mapping of ideas, so we will need a cognitive module. Speech is obviously directed by the rules of language, so we will need a language module. We need to be able to think about what we are saying, so we will need a working memory module to provide awareness. We also need to send driving signals to the speech musculature, so we need a speech output module. These are the obvious modules. But how can we explain any type of disfluency with these?

Not so obvious, we need something such as segmental and suprasegmental modules. Why select those components of spoken language processing and ignore syntactics and semantics, for example? We are indebted for selection of segmental and suprasegmental to Shattuck-Hufnagle (1985), a linguist, for the answer. To account for slips of the tongue she has proposed a convincing theory that these slips could not happen as they do, particularly as they involve transpositions in syllables of equal stress, if speech segments were not assembled separately from the suprasegmental elements of syllable stress. Extending her idea, McNeilage and his colleagues (1985) cast this division of speech assembly labor in the context of a frame-content explanation, for which they proposed an evolutionary lineage, namely, the ability of primates and other lower animals that are capable of holding an object in one hand, the frame, while manipulating it with the other, the content. In speech, they propose that the frame is the syllable with its suprasegmental prosodic elements, the content consists of the articulatory segments that fit within each syllable. So what we have is essentially an assembly line analogy in which speech is assembled from many components from all over the brain.

By assuming that speech output is assembled ultimately from segmental and suprasegmental components, then the final operation must integrate these components before assembly is complete. That being the case, an integrator module is needed. Let us also assume that language processing operations are relatively unavailable to awareness, but that products of the processing are most available, a relatively safe assumption. This is to say that when whatever you are thinking is in verbal form, so that you could speak it or write it, it is in a concise form of which you can be keenly aware. You know what you are saying or are about to say, even though you do not know the grammatic or semantic processes by which you get there when you speak spontaneously. This does not mean you cannot choose words or grammatic constructions deliberately, but when you do you are not speaking spontaneously and self-expressively. This difference points up the most troubling aspect, for me, of using fluency controls for treatment.

Knowing what you want to say implies that you know the order of the segmental elements that will make up the words you are ready to speak, otherwise you would not know the word you are ready to speak. What you are less likely to know are the stresses and intonations you will use, even though they, too are processed simultaneously. Consider why this must be the case. If what you speak is put in writing no information about the syllable, whether stress or any other aspect of prosody, is recorded. The letters tell you only about the sounds. All you need to know to know what you want to say are the segments of the words in proper order. Given these conditions, what we will assume is that when the integrator has selected the segments to produce the word to be spoken, working memory (the awareness module) is notified of readiness to say that word.

On the other side of the integrative process is the suprasegmental input which determines syllable stress involving the prosodic elements of pitch, loudness, and duration. Given that the syllable is the frame within which the appropriate segments must fit, the duration of these segments, then, cannot be determined until duration of the syllable is determined. If you speak slowly, durations of syllables, hence of segments, will be longer than if you speak rapidly. What this means is that the segments cannot be produced until the syllable is available for integration. The syllable is the foundation of the utterance.

Let us consider implications of this arrangement. For example, what would happen if some aspect of linguistic processing were delayed for whatever reason? While searching for the right word or phrase construction the flow of speech would of course be halted one way or another. Because all linguistic processing would have to be completed before the segments for a word could be selected for integration, speakers would experience this disruption as being temporarily halted while they figure out what they are trying to say. This is a process available to awareness, so these disruptions are typically experienced as normal disfluencies, regardless of how they sound.

Now let us reverse the disruption. What would happen if some aspect of suprasegmental processing were delayed relative to segmental processing for any reason? Again speech would be halted one way or another until the syllable frame arrived for integration with its segments. But the integrator does not have access to awareness. Assuming the segments arrived first, their arrival would have notified working memory that you knew what you were ready to say. But working memory receives no information about readiness of the syllable. Without the syllable frame, you would be unable to say the word you are ready to speak for reasons of which you would be unaware. Hence, if you attempted to proceed with what you were ready to say, the resulting disruption would be experienced as involuntary, which by my definition means it would be stuttered.

Since suprasegmental processing of syllable stress is as much a function of language operations as segmental processing, why would suprasegmental processing be delayed? Two possible answers are apparent: the syllable could be delayed in transmission from the language module to the integrator module, and it could be delayed by the integrator in preparing the syllable to receive its segments. Delays for these reasons would presumably be experienced as "stuttering coming out of nowhere." As is often seen in children the blockage would not be anticipated nor be a consequence of emotions. Its effect on the speaker, however, could be just as frustrating, nonetheless.

But chronic stuttering, at least, seems to be fraught with emotion. How is it involved? The modular properties we have so far provide no basis for emotion. But a probable, if not necessary, answer is, for me, the most intriguing part of this explanation. We, along with linguists, have been so preoccupied with language as the human mode of communication that one searches in vain for any mention of our communication origins. I do not mean the origin of speech and language, I mean the origin of human communication. Obviously, animals communicate and our primate cousins still do, so there is no reason to think that our simian ancestors did not also have a mode of communication. There is also no reason to think that we have not preserved that mode. A fundamental precept of evolutionary theory is that no adaptation is ever discarded: it is preserved even if maladaptive. Certainly a communication system is anything but maladaptive, so we must have inherited our ancestral system on which we overlaid our speech and language system.

In what form is that ancient system preserved? I would suggest that human infants, surely, reveal the answer. Their capacity for communicating basic needs is unsurpassed. They leave no ambiguity about how they feel or what they want. They are born with the capacity to communicate essentially the same information that Jane Goodall describes her apes as communicating. When infants babble, what you hear is the melody of human communicating without the segmental notes. What they are unwittingly practicing are the prosodic skills they will need to generate syllabic frames for the segmental content they have yet to discover.

As speech develops they will be able to control the suprasegmental elements of speech long before they will have mastered the segmental elements. Equally, if not more, important, they will retain the ancient ability to communicate how they feel about what they are saying. Eventually, infants will become sufficiently skilled in managing prosody that they will be able to mask what they feel by saying one thing while meaning another. Is it not ironic that it requires skill to do that? They will have two communication systems, one linguistic, the other paralinguistic, operating simultaneously in synchrony when speech flows fluently and spontaneously.

Note that we now have these two systems controlling the same prosodic elements, pitch, loudness and duration. The language module controls suprasegmental syllable stress of the symbol system. The paralinguistic module controls the system for signaling affect and speaker intent. Because both systems use the same vocal elements, the instructions from these two systems must be integrated before the final determination of the pitch, loudness, and duration of a syllable can be made.

The paralinguistic module must somehow accomplish this integration by modulating the suprasegmental output of the language module which determines stress and intonation. That output constrains the suprasegmental modulation possible because word meaning can depend on syllable stress. Consider r-e-c-o-r-d. With stress on the last syllable, reCORD, you made permanent with a verb what you can read or hear with stress on the first syllable, RECord, a noun. So feeling and intent can be signaled vocally only to the extent that word meaning is not distorted. On the other side, the paralinguistic system controls speech rate, for instance, which reflects a speaker's feelings, such as excitement or depression. This would seem to be the foundation on which linguistic prosody is modulated since listeners can hear the same words and know the speaker is excited in one instance and depressed in another. That is, you can speak fast or slow and still preserve syllable stress, which must somehow be determined relative to speaking rate. Thus, the fact that our new symbol system must have been superimposed on our evolutionary signal system suggests that the integrator is sent a syllable frame with integrated signal and symbol system duration values, which since speech flow, a matter solely of durations, is the issue, is the only prosodic value for our concern. We need not worry about pitch or loudness.

Consider the expanded implications now before us. Arrival of the syllable frame at the integrator can now be delayed for emotion signaling reasons as well as suprasegmental symbol system reasons. The effect on speech would be the same: the involuntary disruptions of stuttering.

To understand why emotions, particularly conflict, could delay syllable processing, the Neilsons' concept of neural resources fits nicely. Processing rate depends on neural resources available. The neural resources needed for paralinguistic processing could be selectively depleted relative to segmental resources genetically or by brain injury and stuttering could result. What part of the brain is involved I do not know. They could also be depleted functionally by competition for these resources. What is conflict if not competition? So if the speaker is in conflict over how to speak to an important listener, paralinguistic processing resources could be severely taxed, the result being dyssynchrony of segmental content and syllable frame integration with involuntary blockage a necessary consequence.

This has been an exercise in logic to demonstrate the bare essentials of an explanation that saves the known phenomena of stuttering. It requires a different premise than has been used historically, namely that stuttering is a production problem of the speaker, not a perceptual problem of the listener. What I have not told you yet is that an exploratory study has been done to test this new premise.

Moore (1990) reasoned that since stutterers can tell the difference between faked and real stuttering, even though listeners can not, and can describe the difference as being involuntarily blocked when it is real and not when it is not, then this production experience must be how they detect stuttering. She had a moderately severe life-long stutterer fake her stuttering and then judge recordings of the faked and real stuttering five seconds, one minute, one hour, one day, and four days after the real stuttering occurred. The reasoning was that as the immediate echoic memory of what a particular stutter felt like faded, her accuracy in detecting real from faked stuttering should decline.

To validate the subject's ability to determine which was which, the stutterer was asked to signal anything she considered to be real stuttering. Moore immediately signaled back that she was to complete the word and phrase promptly on which she was disrupted. Then she was to repeat the phrase and fake the stutter. When she did, Moore again signaled her to continue promptly, the assumption being that if it was real she would be unable to continue, if faked then she could continue. On 31 signaled fakes on three different days, she was able to continue, on 35 signaled real stutters she was not. This meant that she was 100% accurate on three different days at knowing whether she had stuttered or not at time of occurrence. When she listened to recordings of the real and faked when contrasted in paired comparisons, her accuracy diminished to 88% five seconds after occurrence, 70% at one minute, 47% at one hour, and 62% thereafter. When she judged faked and real samples separately, her accuracy plummeted close to chance immediately, averaging 56%. Moore also played the same recordings to 18 unsophisticated listeners and their average accuracy was 57%. Since 50% is pure chance, obviously, no one could do anything but guess.

What does this mean? It means that this stutterer could not have relied on auditory perception to detect whether or not she stuttered by her own determination. Not only did she not have enough information in the recordings to judge stuttering accurately, neither did the listeners. It means that listeners have no more certainty whether stuttering has occurred or not than did the children in the apocryphal kindergarten class who determined if their pet hamster was pregnant or not by voting on it. How far this stutterer's results can be generalized to other stutterers of course remains to be determined. At minimum it means that at least one stutterer, probably many judging by Bloodstein and Shogan's similar results with 20 stutterers, and possibly all chronic stutterers determine whether or not they stutter by a production criterion, not a perceptual criterion. If true, it also means that stuttering cannot be a peripheral motor disorder. Since the acoustic signal does not contain the critical information, then the movements that produced that signal also cannot be the problem.

This analysis is about stuttering, not stutterers. The explanation I have laid out does not require that stutterers be different from non-stutterers. They can be, but they need not be, so I do not know the meaning of the statistical, but far from invariant, differences reported between stutterers and nonstutterers. That does not mean there is no connection. It just means I do not know what it is, if it is. And the reason I do not know is because I cannot find a causal connection that logically links differences among stutterers and nonstutterers to all of the phenomena of stuttering that must be explained. My guess is that these differences are not necessary, let alone sufficient, for stuttering.

An observation needs to be added. We have a long tradition of establishing observer reliability by inter- and intrajudge agreement on frequency of stuttering. That is how we have claimed to know that our judges are reasonably accurate. The fact that their agreements are often close to 100% probably has had much to do with preservation of a perceptual definition. After all, how could judges in such high agreement possibly be wrong; and yet here were 18 judges, 19 including the stutterer herself, listening to recordings of her performance, and their accuracy was barely above chance. Only one listener got as high as 68% average accuracy, a far cry from 100%. Yet what they were judging was frequency of occurrence of authentic stuttering, presumably what all judges are attempting to determine when they make their judgments when they have typically been in very high agreement.

Why such a discrepancy when they are all making the same type of judgments? Because historically, observer agreement has been taken as the index of accuracy. But in Moore's study she did something never done before. She developed a procedure for validating the stutterer's judgments of her own stuttering at time of occurrence, so accuracy of all judgments was determined against a validated criterion. Against this criterion, all of these judgments of recorded stuttering were obviously guesses, yet correlations of listener test-retest judgments were close to 0.70 agreement with themselves, which indicated that they were relatively reliably inaccurate. In fact, if all their judgments had been wrong, as the stutterer's were on one occasion, then they would have been 100% in agreement that they were completely wrong.

Admittedly, for experimental purposes the listeners had to make tough comparisons of faked and real stuttering. In real life when judging stuttering, the decisions would have doubtless seemed easier and would probably have been in better agreement. But what Moore's study demonstrated was that no matter how much they agree, they simply do not have the information in the acoustic signal to know for certain that what sounds like stuttering really is stuttering from the stutterer's point of view. Which raises the interesting and troubling question, which we do not have time to pursue: whose problem is this anyway, and for whose benefit do we provide therapy when fluency as judged by clinicians is our objective?

I presented to my colleague, Debora Sue-O'Brien, who does the clinical work which I write about, my conception of why stutterers stutter: if they know what they want to say and can not, that is stuttering. I asked her if this accurately reflected what she had observed. "Yes," she said, "for the most part, but I have seen some who do not know what they are trying to say and still try to push ahead as if they did. They get just as blocked and just as upset about it." It had never occurred to me that time pressure could drive speakers to try to talk when they did not know the word they wanted to say. But that is what Ms. O'Brien described, which yields the necessary conditions for the blockage of what could be called linguistic stuttering.

Does any of this have any clinical significance? I think it does, especially since my recent enlightenment which seems to shed light on the puzzling parallel between language development and stuttering onset and remittance. Both peak at the beginning of school years. Stuttering remittance then continues to puberty at which time about 75% of children thought to stutter will have recovered. Those who have not are almost certain to become chronic.

Now that I have discovered linguistic stuttering, this picture makes sense, at least to me. Remittance of this type of stuttering depends on reduction of at least one of two conditions: time pressure or linguistic uncertainty. The condition that improves as a natural consequence of maturation is, of course, linguistic uncertainty, which probably accounts for most of the 75% recovery. Some linguistic stutterers, however, apparently never acquire sufficient language skills to be free of linguistic uncertainty. When we see these people as adults, they get considerable relief just by raising their awareness of the cause of the problem. If they have only linguistic stuttering, they can then convert involuntary blockage into normal interruptions which may sound like stuttering but no longer feel like stuttering.

The majority of chronic stutterers, however, seem to fit the picture of knowing what they want to say but being unable to say it. We will call this self-expressive stuttering. For them, insight seems to have little effect, so the therapies we currently use are probably about as effective as any on the horizon, which means no cure is in sight. What they point up is the urgency of early detection and prevention, the only hope for cure. As matters now stand, the difficulty in hearing the difference between early disfluency that feels like stuttering from disfluency that merely sounds like stuttering requires erring in favor of over diagnosing. I doubt that anyone will be distressed by having normal disfluency reduced if you over intervene. The price of not intervening when in doubt has the potential consequence of chronic stuttering. That price is too high. So as far as I am concerned, when in doubt clinically, especially with young children, call it stuttering even if it is not.

The essence of what I have attempted to present, from which stem clinical and research implications, is a model of neural functions that would account for my conception of the necessary and sufficient conditions for stuttering.

For stuttering which can and probably does happen to all of us now and then, whether we are disturbed by it or not, the first requirement is for a condition disruptive of the fluent flow of speech. This condition can be any form of linguistic uncertainty for whatever reason, from uncertainty of how to phrase an idea to uncertainty of how to pronounce a word. It can also be reduced neural resources for integrating symbolic stress requirements for prosody with self-expressive emotion-signaling requirements. The depletion of neural resources can be for reason of genetic constraints, brain injury, or conflict (or any other functional condition which reduces paralinguistic neural resources). The important difference in linguistic and self-expressive stuttering is not the disfluency produced but availability of awareness of the cause of the stuttering. The cause of linguistic uncertainty is available to awareness for anyone who chooses to attend, so it can be remedied merely by recognizing that cause. Still, when time pressure drives speech, what starts as normal linguistic disfluency turns into stuttering. The cause of self-expressive stuttering is not available to awareness, however, so it is more profoundly involuntary, hence resistant to remediation, let alone cure.

Stuttering that persists as a chronic problem for the speaker and leads to an identity of being a stutterer requires a second condition: time pressure. Without it, the urgency to proceed with an utterance despite being involuntarily blocked would not exist. A speaker would be able to do what one normally does when disrupted, stop until you are able to proceed, with possibly some nonverbal filler tossed in to hold your place in the conversation. Because the self-expressive stutterer knows what he is trying to say, the fact that he can not is particularly perplexing and frustrating, so he is probably most likely to become vulnerable to time pressure, and eventually to chronic stuttering.

This explanation I have presented is not just my conception. It is the work of three others in addition to myself: Dick Curlee, Ray Kent, and Tom Hixon. It has been evolving for about a decade. The reason it is presented now is because we finally reached the point where our revisions were simply more cosmetic than substantive. Until Ms. O'Brien enlightened me about linguistic stuttering, we knew in the back of our minds that the language role in stuttering would probably need revision, but after years of living with that issue, we could find no explanation except that delays in language processing produce nonstuttered disfluency, which is probably true most of the time, but as Ms. O'Brien pointed out, not always.

We have no illusions that this is the final word, but more likely it is probably equivalent to the map Columbus thought would take him to India. We hope we are headed in the right direction.

References

Bloom, L. and Beckwith, R. (1989). Talking with feeling: Integrating affective and linguistic expression in early language development. *Cognition and Emotion* 3: 313–42.

Guitar, B., Guitar, C., Neilson, P., O'Dwyer, N. and Andrews, G. (1988). Onset sequencing of selected lip muscles in stutterers and nonstutterers. *Journal of Speech and Hearing Research* 31: 28–35.

Kelly, E. and Conture, E. (1988). Acoustic and perceptual correlates of typical and imitated stuttering. *Journal of Fluency Disorders* 13: 232–52.

Kent, R. (1985). Developing and disordered speech: Strategies for organization. *American Speech-Language-Hearing Association Report #15* 6: 29–37.

MacNeilage, P., Studdert-Kennedy, M. and Lindblom, B. (1985). Planning and production of speech: An overview. *American Speech-Language-Hearing Association Report #15* 4: 15–21.

Moore, S. and Perkins, W.H. (1990). Validity and reliability of judgements of authentic and simulated stuttering. *Journal of Speech and Hearing Disorders* 55: 383–91

Perkins, W., Kent, R. and Curlee, R. (1991). A theory of neuropsycholinguistic functions in stuttering. *Journal of Speech and Hearing Research* 34: 734–52.

Schwartz, H. and Conture, E. (1988). Subgrouping young stutterers: Preliminary behavioral observations. *Journal of Speech and Hearing Research* 31: 62–71.

Shattuck-Hufnagel, S. (1985). Context similarity constraints on segmental speech errors: An experimental investigation of the role of word position and lexical stress. *American Speech-Language-Hearing Association Report #15* 8: 43–49.

Discussion

K. Burk: This conference has been an exciting interaction; an international, national, and local kind of interaction. Bill did an excellent job of presenting and I would like to express our appreciation to him for building a theory for us and inviting target practice. We do have some questions and comments from my group that I would like to share. First of all, it was viewed as a very positive thing to once again look at stuttering as it is defined by the stutterer. This is not always done. Another comment had to do with the theory seeming to fit the incipient stutterer a little bit more closely perhaps than the confirmed stutterer. The theory itself, however, was viewed, in some respects, as not really reflecting all the available empirical data. There are data that seem not to have been reflected in the theory. Maybe we could get at that by asking Dr. Perkins the question, "if we were to generate a series of research directions, how would the theory be tested?" Is it testable as stated?

Editor's Note

Following the conference Dr. Perkins submitted what he felt was a more satisfactory response to Dr. Burk's first question. His revised response is included here. During his conference presentation Dr. Perkins presented a visual model and referred to it during his talk. Since that model was included in a paper submitted for publication elsewhere it could not be included here. Therefore, questions and discussion relating specifically to that model have been deleted from this discussion section. The model appears in: Perkins, W., Kent, R. and Curlee, R. (1991). A theory of neuropsycholinguistic function in stuttering. *Journal of Speech and Hearing Research.* Other references cited in the paper or in the discussion can be found at the end of the paper.

W. Perkins: The question was asked, how can this theory be tested. The theory presented accounts for stuttering, not stutterers. Any phenomena of stuttering constitute a test. To the extent that any credible evidence about stuttering cannot be explained, then to that extent the theory is wrong.

Since the theory was formulated, a few recent studies have constituted such a test. Bloom and Beckwith (1989) have shown that affective and linguistic expression systems develop independently and are eventually integrated, which is congruent with the paralinguistic/segmental division of processing for spoken language. Kelly and Conture (1988) could find no acoustic differences between faked and real stuttering, which supports the basic conception of this theory that stuttering is a production rather than a perceptual disorder. Similarly, Guitar and colleagues (1987) found lip innervation evidence of involuntary blockage in stuttering. Supporting the aspect of the theory that topography of stuttering varies along a continuum of articulatory effort, Schwartz and Conture (1988) report that only a few of the young stutterers they studied produced one type of stuttering.

The theory was constructed to account for the necessary and sufficient neural functions required for stuttering. As such it makes no predictions about the neural sites of these functions. What it does predict is that each module involves discrete neural activity that can, potentially, be detected. As equipment becomes available to detect these rapidly changing activities, their locations in the brain should become evident as the behavioral components of stuttering are varied systematically. An appropriate experiment to begin with would be an investigation of the difference in neural activity between authentic and simulated stuttering. Because one type of disfluency feels like stuttering and the other does not, even though they both sound alike, the neural difference between them would define the boundaries of the essential neurology of stuttering. Within those boundaries should be found evidence of the activity of the neural modules hypothesized to be involved in stuttering.

A. Rochet: I also convey appreciation from my group for your and Dr. Ingham's emphasis on acknowledging the stutterer's complaint and on utilizing the stutterer's validations of moments of stuttering and encouraging their inclusion in operational definitions of the problem. With respect to that, some people wish that you would clarify further what you are advocating with respect to using the stutterers' information in measuring or describing stuttering, especially where there may be a discrepancy between what the clinician perceives and what the client perceives. How narrow is your definition of using this?

W. Perkins: Let me begin by saying that it seems to me that the big responsibility that we should be looking at as our primary task is prevention of the development of chronic stuttering. Anything we can do to achieve that would make our profession worthwhile, all by itself. So from the standpoint of early detection and intervention, and doing all that can be done to prevent the development of stuttering, I do not see differentiation between stuttering as perceived by the stutterer and stuttering as perceived by the listener, I do not see that as being a terribly crucial issue. In fact, I would err in favour of letting anything that even gives you a suspicion that they are stuttering be the basis for early intervention, with any good prevention operations you can perform. So when in doubt, intervene, whether it really is stuttering or whether it is not. The place that this distinction between stuttering perceived by the stutterer and stuttering perceived by the listener comes in, is mainly in terms of the kinds of adult treatment programs and adolescent treatment programs that we use. If we concentrate on listener identification of stuttering then we tend to set up our own ideas as to what is the proper fluency performance and what is not. We have become the administrators of therapeutic goals, in effect. By our setting fluency as the goal, this then becomes the goal for treatment. I am not sure, and I am personally not at all persuaded, that fluency is a desirable goal, let alone an appropriate goal. The main reason I am really concerned about it as an appropriate goal is because fluency, when it is managed by the clinician, particularly if the clinician uses extrinsic reinforcement to maintain that fluency, can very easily lead to a clinically sanctioned avoidance operation. And if there is one thing that is like having a cancer that has not been removed, it is avoidance. So even though procedurally this distinction does not really change much in terms of what we do, for me at least it changes why I am doing it and what my objectives are in doing the things I do.

A. Rochet: Some among us perceived a possible categorical difference between your "linguistic uncertainty" group of speakers and your "self-expressive" stuttering group of speakers. How does your conceptualization of these two groups handle a problem where fluency shaping helps the "self-expressive" stutterer to evolve into a "linguistically uncertain" stutterer (because of his limited linguistic practice), but one who can still experience the involuntary losses of self-control that constitute real stuttering?

W. Perkins: Since I have just discovered "linguistic stuttering" I have not thought about it as long as I have about "self-expressive" stuttering. But quite clearly, what little I have thought about it and what little information I have on it, I would agree. I think they are two categorically different sets of problems but they interact in almost every case that we have encountered. They interact most of the time. Rarely do you find a pure "linguistic" stutterer at the adolescent or adult level. Most of them are likely to have recovered in that early recovery period.

With adults we do find quite a few who are not certain of what they are trying to say. That in itself produces a lot of disfluency. They all show time pressure. If you take time pressure out of the equation, I think you would not get stuttering under any of these conditions. You can have involuntary blockage, that by definition is stuttering, but does not constitute a problem. What you hear me going through much of the time involves what I think, quite literally, can be called involuntary blockage because I am stopped in trying to go forward. But I do not feel under the kind of pressure that would force me to try and push through it, in ways that I feel like I have been tripped. We had one very severe stutterer who got out about one sylla-ble per 20 seconds. We put him on DAF. With this fellow we started out down at the 200 millisecond rate and he was going along -l-i-i-k-e t-h-i-i-s. After a week of this, we would normally have gotten him down to the 150 rate. When we cut it back to 150 rate he w-a-a-s s-t—i—ll going along at the 200 rate. We cut it back to 100, he was st-i-i-ll going along at the 200 rate. We cut the whole thing off and he was st - - i-i-ll going along at that 200 rate. Finally, we asked him, "doesn't that seem slow to you?" His reply was, "no-o-, it'ssss toooo fastttt?" I am sure, he had been speaking this way for so long that he had no skills to put larger units together and speak fluently with ideas as his cen-tral theme. He just did not have the practice of dealing with anything but o—n—e syllable at a time. Before he found DAF, he would be stuck for 20 seconds or more, then go on to the next syllable. His communication with DAF seemed awfully tortuous, but it was faster than he went when he stuttered.

M. Neilson: My group zeroed in on just one thing—this whole con-cept of a difference between "self-expressive" stuttering and "linguistic" stuttering. Had you been there Bill, you would have received strong endorsement for the fact that these seem to be qualitatively different things. In terms of do they both exist in the same stutterer? We said "he is going to say yes." Are they represented in different proportions, in different situ-ations, at different development stages? I said that you were going to say yes. Therefore, since I have answered the question for you, and since you gave me an invitation, I would like to answer you in terms of the sorts of thinking that Peter Neilson and I have been doing about neural resources. I cannot possibly hope to put that model to the audience in the couple of minutes that I am stealing. One of the tenets, I suppose, of our way of thinking about stuttering is in terms of basic inefficiency of certain neural resources. We would see that as being based at the speech motor control end. In order words, it would contribute to "self-expressive" stuttering, as you said. But in order to account for much that we know about the variability of stuttering (both in terms of the linguistic loci, the variability across different situations and the fluency inducing conditions), it seems to me that we have to postulate that there is some sharing of linguistic resources and speech motor control processing resources. That is a central feature of the way we are now thinking about stuttering. Of course, that fits very nicely into the capacities and demands framework. I was delighted that Woody Starkweather took that up and ran with it. It was an idea that we planted in embryonic form at ASHA in 1981, when Gavin Andrews presented a mini-seminar which eventually became that big paper in *JSHD*. That was the crucial idea—that if you do not have enough processing space you may steal some processing that was to be assigned elsewhere i.e., linguistically.

W. Perkins: As far as I can see, you have got to pull this speech motor assembly operation apart so that you have a linguistic part and a nonlinguistic part that have to be assembled in order to account for all the different things, particularly the way emotion figures into the stuttering that you find in chronic stutterers.

M. Neilson: Our ways of putting things on the surface look rather different. I am beginning to think that they are perhaps much closer than we initially thought. I would like to come back to your concepts about emotional involuntariness but we did have another question in the group. That was, between "self-expressive" stuttering and "linguistic" stuttering. Do you have suggestions for a formal way in which these might be distinguished by the clinician working at the coal face? Once again, we are back to the "what I do on Monday morning" problem. People were asking whether clinicians can distinguish these objectively. Can they work on both? Can or should they work on both the linguistic aspects and the self-expressive aspects of stuttering at the same time?

W. Perkins: I think they can. I do not know of any operational definition to differentiate them that does not involve a subjective response so we just simply ask them. "Did you know what you were trying to say when you had that stutter?" Most of them say "yes" but some of them say "no." When they say "no," we start helping them be aware of their linguistic indecisions, their linguistic uncertainty as the basis for much of what is disrupting them. You see, you get a disruption in the flow of speech just as well when you have a delay in the segmental input as when you have a delay in syllabic input. It is like the assembly line for putting the motor in the chassis. If the motor does not arrive, the chassis does not have much chance to move. If the motor arrives and the chassis does not, you are not going to get it off the assembly line either. Either way you are going to get speech disruption. But the linguistic operation is available to awareness, and it is readily available to awareness. So with adults, who have little skill in assembling their language into larger units, I think a very appropriate thing to do with them is to work as if it were a language problem, trying to assemble their ideas into larger units of expression.

M. Neilson: You mean like when I yell at the people in my group program—"don't open your mouth until you know what you want to say?"

W. Perkins: Yes. But those who do know what they want to say and cannot, those are the ones that I am calling "self-expressive" stutterers. As far as minimizing the disruptive effects of linguistic uncertainty, I would agree with your idea of helping them to be aware that if they do open their mouths and try to talk before they know what they are trying to say, they are inviting stuttering.

M. Neilson: I should have prefaced that by pointing out that I only say that after they have gone through a fluency induction and I know that they are capable of saying anything that they want to say. Sometimes it is just that they have not worked out what they want to say. When they have stopped and I yell at them for stopping inappropriately, they say, "It's okay that I stopped, I was just thinking of the word." Then I say, that is where you have to pay special attention to the fluency skills because when you are just thinking of the word, you are just retrieving something recalcitrant from your lexicon. You are doing a lot of linguistic processing which means that it is comprising whatever is left over to subserve fluency. That is especially where you have to pay attention. Therefore when someone stops before a word, I would not let them get away with saying "I only stopped because I was thinking of the word." Right? One more thing. Faked versus real stuttering? The data from Dr. Moore that you alluded to is fascinating. You are really saying that the difference is in the involuntary act, I think.

And you seem to be saying that involuntariness is something that reaches awareness after the fact. In other words, it happens and then you become aware it is happening. You are not aware that it is going to happen. Would that be right?

W. Perkins: I suspect that people can get an aura of difficulty. What is experienced when you anticipate stuttering I am not sure, because I have never felt that. I am certainly disfluent in ways that sound like stuttering to a lot of people, including a lot of stutterers, but I do not know what the feeling of anticipation of stuttering is. I would suspect that one way or another you have an anticipation. Possibly it is just your history of knowing that you are going to have trouble with certain words and certain sounds, that you are going to lose control of them. That may be sufficient to provide the basis for that anticipation without necessarily having any access to awareness of the delayed suprasegmental input to the integrator.

M. Neilson: Let me explain where I am coming from and the way that we conceptualize stuttering. A key feature is the involuntariness of it. The way I like to think about it is in terms of these inefficient neural resources that are subserving the sensory motor integration process, which is the foundation for, in fact, being able to pull out any set of motor commands to fulfill a set of expected sensory consequences that you know that you want to produce.

First of all you have to know what it is you are going to have to sound like. I am not talking about linguistic formulation here. I am really talking about the phonetic trajectory that you are going to have to follow. Now it seems that if you had inefficient resources in that sort of translation, you may well know what it is going to sound like, but because the translation did not happen properly, partly because you did not have the resources or did not allocate them properly, you would end up with something you did not expect.

Let me give you an analogy. Remember that big blackout that occurred in the whole northeastern part of the United States many years ago? There was a story, perhaps apocryphal, of a lady who repaired her iron. Her husband had been asked to do it for several weeks but he had not done it, so she just sat down and repaired it herself. She then put in the plug to start ironing and the whole of the northeastern states blacked out. That was a sensory consequence which she did not expect! She did not have any control of it, but she felt that she had done it. Ever put your foot on the brake in a car and expect it to slow down and it did not? You know what you expected to happen. It did not happen. In that circumstance your attention gets very highly focused on what is happening to you. The particular concept of stuttering that we have says that when a person stutters, certainly with self-expressive type stuttering, he is in a circumstance where the expected sensory consequence does not match up with what actually happens. You do not feel that you did it. You feel that it got done to you. It happened, it was outside your control, and that is my definition of involuntariness.

W. Perkins: Well, I have not had a chance to think that one through. I think the people who can validate it are the people who stutter.

M. Neilson: Finally, I want to say, as the one who has come the farthest to this conference, that it is a very special experience for me, to be in a room full of people all of whom are focused on this disorder. It is unusual. You certainly could not do it in Australia. I expect it does not often happen in North America, that you can have a group of people, of this size, focused for this length of time, all discussing this fascinating disorder. I think this Banff conference has been really wonderful, especially from my point of view.

L. Manz: I would like to thank our speaker Dr. Perkins and our discussion leaders, Ken Burk, Anne Rochet, and Megan Neilson for a job well done. I would like once again to extend a sincere thanks to Dr. Boberg. Not just for the conference but for the years of planning and preparation that have gone into organizing it.

Epilogue

To provide another perspective on the conference the Editor invited the discussion leaders, twenty months after the conference, to reflect on the material presented and discussed at the conference. Specifically, they were asked to share their general observations and reactions to the debate over whether there were implications for assessment and therapy in the material presented at the conference and what the focus of future research might be. Submissions were received from Dr. Anne Rochet, Dr. Hugo Gregory and Dr. Megan Neilson.

Anne Rochet

My perspective, as participant and discussion leader, at the 1989 Banff Conference was that of a student of motor speech disorders, in general. A major component of my clinical and research interests includes the instrumental assessment of aeromechanical, biomechanical and acoustical parameters of normal and dysarthric speech production. Therefore, although I do not have a professional history of involvement in stuttering research and treatment, per se, the concept of stuttering as a motor control disorder has kept me interested in the evolution of efforts to investigate disfluency from neuropsychological and neurophysiological perspectives. Admittedly, my reactions to the conference presentations and discussion that they generated were influenced by my own biases about models of speech motor control, and limited by my ignorance of the current literature on stuttering. Therefore, I relied on the premise that the principles of experimental design and behaviour measurement and analysis are universal to the critical appraisal of research in any aspect of speech production and used these principles as a basis from which to listen, understand and question at the Conference.

Dr. Mateer's place as first on the program set the stage appropriately for an appreciation of the myriad of ontogenetic neurochemical, developmental, maturational, environmental and psychoemotional factors that could contribute to a disruption of coordinative and sequential voluntary motor behaviours that constitute fluent speech. Her review also served to emphasize that these factors contribute to the heterogeneity among persons who stutter with respect to possible causes for the onset and maintenance of disfluency.

Dr. Moore's historical review of neurophysiological assessment phenomena traced the evolution of a number of imaging, perceptual and electrophysiological tests whereby one can attempt to observe differences in cerebral hemispheric processing among individuals performing various cognitive tasks. He noted that these windows on neurophysiological processes are fraught with some ambiguity, however, because the cognitive processes they reflect are multidimensional, and differences may be observable or obscured depending upon the cognitive mode of information processing in which the subject is operating. It seemed to be understood, on the basis of his presentation as well as his comments during the subsequent discussion of it, that we cannot yet assume a cause and effect relationship between the neurophysiological phenomena and the coincident behavior he measures that is sufficient to serve as a criterion of diagnostic or prognostic accuracy or treatment efficacy for disfluent speech without more careful (and carefully replicated) experimentation.

Dr. Webster's presentation was illustrated by the experimental data he has collected on unimodal and bimodal oral and manual motor tasks that imply a basic instability in, or among, certain components of the central nervous system in stutterers (specifically the supplementary motor area, the corpus callosum and right cerebral hemisphere). His data begin to provide tangible evidence for a basic neurophysiological anomaly in adult stutterers that deserves further investigation, although the data do not prove that the anomaly causes stuttering or goes away when the stutterer is not stuttering, or that treatment is successful if it teaches compensatory behaviors for the fragile motor control anomaly. He was careful to call the model he presented speculative, particularly with respect to the effects of fluency shaping and desensitization treatment on the basic anomaly, and suggested experiments that needed to be done to support his hypotheses.

Finally, the cluster analyses of Dr. Yeudall and his colleagues highlighted the multiple sources of variability within the neuropsychological profiles of the stutterers they studied that might be responsible in part, or in concert with other factors, for stuttered versus fluent speech. Their data implicated not only the regions cited by Mateer, Moore and Webster as potential sites for speech motor control breakdown, but also possible, the midbrain, thalamus and brain stem.

These presentations that constituted the invited technical paper components of the Conference were interesting and provocative, as the transcripts of their discussion periods show. Nevertheless, to this observer at least, they also made it clear that there were as yet very limited neurophysiological and neuropsychological data bases from which to infer extensively about diagnosis, prognosis and treatment for stuttering. Therefore, it was not surprising that the reviews of Dr. Curlee and Dr. Ingham exposed those limitations, nor was it surprising that many found the exposure threatening. In my opinion, however, the debate they provoked was valuable for several reasons.

Curlee and Ingham resisted the temptation for and the pitfalls of unbridled inference. An elaboration of implications presumes that some kind of functional relationship has been inferred to exist among the neuropsychological theories presented, the data obtained thus far and stuttering. No presentation at the Conference demonstrated that, however, Mateer reviewed the factors that could conspire to disrupt fluency. Moore reviewed the multidimensional neurophysiological recording/imaging techniques that might reveal that disruption, and Yeudall et al. the neuropsychological performance variables that may reflect neurophysiological instability. Webster reviewed some experimental models that might be applied fruitfully to more specific correlative questions about oral and manual motor performance vis-a-vis changes in speech fluency effected by different types of stuttering treatment. To infer extensively from the papers and data presented, however, farther than the presenters themselves did, to any or all other aspects of assessment and treatment of stuttering would have been an exercise in speculation.

Extensive discussions of implications tend to be self-serving and self-satisfying. As such, they serve to mask, to some extent, gaps or even chasms in an inferential data base. In this regard, the critical reviews of Curlee and Ingham also were valuable in that they revealed the areas where implication was illegitimate because there was not relevant data from which to generalize or because measurement limitations restricted experimental explorations. One of Curlee's most potent points was that although the neurophysiological research conducted thus far does appear to elucidate neurological correlates of stuttered speech behavior, it has yet to isolate or designate which among the many factors are true correlates, predictors or provocative agents of stuttering and which are merely coincident phenomena. Furthermore, he argued logically that the information summarized at the Conference is still a long way from being able to shed light on some of the most difficult and elusive aspects of day-to-day problem-solving with respect to stuttering diagnosis, treatment and prognosis, particularly in children.

Ingham expressed major concern about several issues that can compromise current and future research: a lack of consistently-applied operational definitions of phenomena such as natural fluency, contrived fluency, natural stuttering and controlled stuttering, among others; relative ignorance about the variables influencing the perception and production of the locus of control in stuttering; and poor reliability among observers of stuttering moments and between observers and producers of stuttering behavior. The good credentials and intentions of many researchers notwithstanding, the targets of Ingham's concern are threats to the internal and external validity of clinical research on any aspect of the assessment and treatment of stuttering (or dyspraxia or dysarthria), and their resolution is crucial to the credibility and reliability of results obtained and their use as a basis for further investigation.

It seems to me that every discipline needs the introspective "conscience" that the Curlee and Ingham papers provided at this Conference . . . a self-critical, peer-review that constitutes a healthy threat to self-assurance or "tunnel-vision," and therefore serves as a potent stimulus for self-criticism, re-evaluation of the research that has been done and careful assessment of that which still needs to be done. From my perspective, their observations provided a realistic assessment of the Conference: namely, that the viewpoints and data presented had brought the participants to a threshold from which a number of compelling research avenues extending into the future became apparent. As the opportunity for this valuable Conference arises again in 1994, perhaps it would be productive to charge each presenter with devoting a certain portion of his or her paper to the experimentation required to test, validate, replicate or extend the models, hypotheses or empirical results presented. In this way, the intellectual energies of the conferees would be devoted less to inference and more to reaching a consensus on and even drafting some of the necessary research questions that will make the five years between conferences productive on a number of fronts.

Hugo Gregory

Findings about brain hemispheric functioning in adult stutterers, including changes that occur during therapy, support what most clinicians do in therapy that has been observed as successful. In addition, this research helps us understand why rather long-term follow-up (maintenance) is necessary.

Techniques for modifying rate, speech initiation, coarticulation, blending, inflection, and pausing seem appropriate in terms of strengthening left hemispheric control of the temporal-segmental aspects of speech production. Relaxation procedures and desensitization approaches, that deal more specifically with negative emotion, are appropriate for reducing right hemispheric interference with the left hemisphere's dominant role in speech production. This brain functioning perspective gives added insight into the long-term nature of the therapy process. The stabilization of changes in behavior and brain functioning takes time.

There are individual differences in neural control of speech. Therefore, residual stuttering may be due to some extent to the person possessing less capacity for the production of fluent speech. Finally, this research reminds us of the many factors (e.g., linguistic, motor, and emotional) that should be considered in therapy.

Megan D. Neilson

As an epilogue to the conference proceedings Dr. Boberg has asked discussion leaders to comment on what he has described as the "spirited and healthy debate, in the best scientific tradition, on whether there were any implications for diagnosis and therapy in the research papers presented at the conference." He has also asked for some reflections on where research efforts might be focused in the near future. Rather than deal separately with these briefs I have chosen to offer some thoughts as to how a new neurobiological research trend, as yet only looming on the horizon in regard to stuttering, may eventually help to defuse the need for such fervent debate. First though, such argument seems to be inevitable in the path to understanding many clinical disorders. Most saliently, we should note how dissent readily dissipates once basic research provides the key to the nature of the disorder. Thus research on the cause of schizophrenia can still engender acrimony from those concerned with its clinical management, whereas the worth of elucidating the mechanisms underlying diabetes now goes unquestioned.

The latter part of the 1980s saw rapid burgeoning of what is known variously as "connectionism," "neural networks," or "computational neuroscience" (Sejnowski, Koch and Churchland, 1988). The province of this field overlaps with longer established areas such as artificial intelligence, linguistics, cognitive neuroscience, robotics and adaptive control. The link occurs because each of these areas involves the development of computational systems which can emulate or "model" the behavior of a biological or technological process. Formerly this has been accomplished in various ways according to the traditions of the various disciplines. This is now beginning to be accomplished in common across the fields by using multilayered networks of interconnected elements in which the influence of one element on another is adjusted iteratively until a satisfactory model is achieved. The fact that these computational systems "learn," plus their diagrammatic likeness to interconnected "cells," leads easily to the label "neural networks." Unfortunately this term can mislead because many such networks, while computationally satisfactory in modeling a cognitive or neurobiological process, achieve this by mechanisms which are not biologically feasible, the most common being "backpropagation." While such models are interesting in their own right and useful in many applications, it is those developed in light of realistic neurological structure and function which promise most to neuroscience. This is the new area which I believe can greatly influence our understanding of cognitive and sensorimotor control processes and be especially relevant in the study of language/speech and its disorders.

Our own beginnings in the application of computational neuroscience principles to sensorimotor control are found in Neilson and Neilson (1987) and we have recently extended this in Neilson, Neilson and O'Dwyer (1992). Detail is not appropriate here but in summary, we propose a computational model, consistent with established neural structure and function, which emulates adaptive sensorimotor behavior. A fundamental feature of this, and indeed most neural network models, is its inherent parallel distributed processing (PDP) architecture. The whole concept of PDP systems, biologically based or not, is seductively "brain-like," which leads to an important further analogy. The notion of computational modules operating in parallel rather than sequentially fits neatly with the conceptualization of neural resources which may be allocated in greater or lesser amounts to a particular stage of a particular task. This resources framework leads us directly to the concepts of capacity and demand now firmly established in the cognitive/behavioral literature (see Navon and Gopher, 1979) and used by ourselves and Starkweather and his associates in relation to stuttering and the amelioration of disfluency (see Adams, 1990). This forges the link that I foresee between a computational neuroscience formulation of stuttering and future implications for diagnosis and treatment.

There are multiple ways in which a computational PDP model of the language/speech production system, in whole or in part, may be helpful. One strategy with good face validity in regard to eventual treatment benefit is to use such a model to explore the characteristics of speech/accuracy performance tradeoff. Also feasible is the exploration of these characteristics in a model where allocation of resources is modulated by an "attentional" process. The role of attention is just beginning to be addressed in terms of PDP models (Cohen, Dunbar and McClelland, 1990) and in stuttering the well-known operant studies pointed clearly to the relevance of this factor long ago. But perhaps the most rewarding use of computational models will be in examining the interplan and potential overlap between processing resources which subserve linguistic formulation and speech motor control. Here I can draw directly on what transpired at Banff. Catherine Mateer presented data indicative of language/speech overlap in some sections of cortex, leading to the suggestion that stuttering may possibly involve language dysfunction. This interplay between language/speech processes was subsequently endorsed by several other speakers as well as in the discussion sessions, and indeed the conference closed with all of us contemplating Bill Perkins's "linguistic stuttering" and "self-expressive stuttering." Language/speech interaction has always been an intrinsic part of the demands and capacities formulation of stuttering (see Andrews et al., 1983; Starkweather, 1987) and relevant evidence has been concisely documented recently by Peters and Starkweather (1990).

I am very hopeful that the foreseeable future will bring the development of biologically based computational models of the interconnected processes that comprise linguistic formulation and speech motor production. Already the recent Nijmegen meeting has seen the presentation of a connectionist model of linguistic processing (Dell, 1991), followed quite independently by a network model of speech motor control (Saltzman, 1991) and the potential complementarity was much remarked upon. An eventually wholistic model will necessarily involve multiple transformations between multiple language/speech process levels. Its complexity may be daunting, but its skeleton should simplify to something close to the levels of representation we recognize today. Computational neuroscience can provide us with a quantitative description of the steps between those levels. These tools will allow us to characterize normal functioning in a way not previously possible and will in turn allow us to impede or enhance various processing steps to determine the sources of breakdown behaviors. Here we can manipulate the limits of neural capacity and demand in a way not possible in the real system yet obtain results that will be directly testable in the clinic in terms of diagnostic and treatment relevance.

References

Adams, M.R. (1990). The demands and capacities model I: Theoretical elaborations. *Journal of Fluency Disorders* 15: 135–41.

Andrews, G., Craig, A., Feyer, A.M., Hoddinott, S., Howie, P. and Neilson, M. (1983). Stuttering: A review of research findings and theories circa 1982. *Journal of Speech and Hearing Disorders* 48: 226–46.

Cohen, J.D., Dunbar, K. and McClelland, J.L. (1990). On the control of automatic processes: A parallel distributed processing model of the Stroop effect. *Psychological Review* 97: 332–61

Dell, G.S. (1991). Connectionist approaches to the production of words. In H.F.M. Peters, W. Hulstijn and C.W. Starkweather, eds., *Speech motor control and stuttering*. Amsterdam: Elsevier.

Navon, D. and Gopher, D. (1979). On the economy of the human-processing system. *Psychological Review* 86: 214–55.

Neilson, M.D., and Neilson, P.D. (1987). Speech motor control and stuttering. *Speech Communication* 6: 325–33.

Neilson, P.D., Neilson, M.D. and O'Dwyer, N.J. (1992). Adaptive model theory: Application to disorders of motor control. In J.J. Summers, ed., *Approaches to the study of motor control and learning (Advances in Psychology Series)*. Amsterdam: North-Holland.

Peters, H.F.M. and Starkweather, C.W. (1990). The interaction between speech motor coordination and language processes in the development of stuttering. *Journal of Fluency Disorders* 15: 115–25.

Saltzman, E. (1991). The task dynamic model in speech production. In H.F.M. Peters, W. Hulstijn and C.W. Starkweather, eds., *Speech motor control and stuttering*. Amsterdam: Elsevier.

Sejnowski, T.J., Koch, C. and Churchland, P.S. (1988). Computational neuroscience. *Science* 241: 1299–1306.

Starkweather, C.W. (1987). *Fluency and Stuttering*. Englewood Cliffs, NJ: Prentice-Hall.